Stories of Chronic Illness, Disability, Healing and Life

My Body of Knowledge

Including:
Crohn's Disease
CFIDS • AIDS • RSI
Muscular Dystrophy
Lyme Disease
Multiple Sclerosis
and Cancer

Edited by
Karen Myers and Felicia Ferlin

Cracked Bell Publishing
San Francisco, California

Cover Illustration by Felicia Ferlin

Published by:
Cracked Bell Publishing
San Francisco, CA 94122
Email: CrackedBell@sbcglobal.net

Library of Congress Cataloging-in-Publication Data
My Body of Knowledge : Stories of Chronic Illness, Disability, Healing and Life / edited by Karen Myers and Felicia Ferlin.
p. cm. Includes bibliographical references.
I. Sick in literature. II. People with disabilities, Writings of, American. III. People with disabilities—United States—Literary collections.
ISBN 978-0-9818172-4-8 2008906052

This book is dedicated to

everyone who lives with a chronic illness or disability, and to those who want to better understand our experience.

Contents

Chapter Four: Interaction, Negotiation, and Relationships

Chapter Five: Integration, Distraction, and Recreation

Ring the bells that still can ring.
Forget your perfect offering.
There is a crack in everything.
That's how the light gets in.

–Leonard Cohen, "Anthem"

Introduction

We all walk along a shifting continuum between health and illness. Some of us are robust and athletic. Some of us undergo surgery or experience cancer. Some of us are born with, or develop, chronic, debilitating conditions.

Those on the "healthy" side of the continuum sometimes can't relate to those with severe disabilities. Those who are experiencing illness sometimes feel separate from and misunderstood by the healthy folks. We create categories to label ourselves and each other. Judgments and stereotypes emerge.

Even those of us who have entered the realm of "ailing health" sometimes distance ourselves from each other, getting lost in the language of disease. When Felicia and I first sought out contributors to this anthology, some people didn't want to submit writing because they didn't consider themselves to be "disabled." They had "a condition" or were "injured."

The writing in this book comes from people with chronic physical conditions, whether you call them injuries, illnesses, disabilities, or diseases. The intent of this book is to share our experiences of living in a human body and to help us reconnect with each other.

Felicia and I created *My Body of Knowledge* in response to our own feelings of isolation and frustration as we dealt with the complex physical and emotional challenges brought on by our disabilities. I have FSH, a form of muscular dystrophy; Felicia has thoracic outlet syndrome, a repetitive strain injury that restricts blood flow and causes painful compression of the nerves. We are in our early 40s and living lives we never would have predicted when we were younger, stronger, and thought we were invincible. But, our bodies took us on paths different from the ones we had envisioned for ourselves.

We had both read many books and articles about people with disabilities, and we found very little writing we could relate to. I do not use a wheelchair, as most people assume when they hear the words muscular dystrophy. Because Felicia's disability is invisible, she is perceived as being healthy, but she can sit for only short periods of time and relies on modifications to keep from experiencing a flare-up.

We noticed people with disabilities were often portrayed as superhuman, overcoming insurmountable obstacles. Where were all the stories about the regular tribulations of life with disease? Are we still valuable and worthwhile on the days when we lie on the sofa overwhelmed by fatigue or hopelessness? Must we always be inspirational and positive?

We realized how many pieces are written *about* people with disabilities, rather than *by* people with disabilities. While these stories have their own merit, we weren't finding them personally helpful. How I am viewed by my family members, friends, and acquaintances does not always reflect what I am experiencing inside. Grief and fear and rage hide beneath the surface.

My Body of Knowledge illustrates the full spectrum of life with a disease or a disability—how sex becomes creative when one is having leg spasms from cerebral palsy, how mundane it is to spend the afternoon staring out the window while recuperating from a painful abdominal surgery, how annoying strangers can be when they don't know how to respond to our disabilities. It delves into the depths of despair and comes back up to the lightness of laughter. It shows that we can experience sorrow and spiritual breakthroughs as readily as we can break into an Elvis impersonation or realize "I can't go on a spiritual journey—I'm constipated."

My Body of Knowledge spotlights 34 writers with a variety of illnesses and disabilities, writing styles, and perspectives. Comprised of five chapters, it begins with stories of initial diagnosis and crisis. It explores how we sometimes withdraw from others and feel alienated as our bodies demand all of our attention. Writers share how their illnesses led them towards profound places of self-reflection and spirituality. They examine how their disabilities affect their relationships with their families, friends, lovers, and strangers. The book concludes with writing in which disability has become integrated with everyday happenings and is merely a backdrop to the richness of life.

This book isn't a how-to manual. It will not teach you ways to cure an illness or eliminate pain. It is simply an expression of the human experience. It shares some insights into how it feels to live in a body that may not be cooperating as well as we had hoped. It weaves together the experience of disability and humanness, exploring life in all its complexity.

I am grateful to all of the writers who were kind enough to share their words and allow us a glimpse into their worlds. Thank you for bringing to light some of the things we don't often say out loud.

We hope you enjoy our collective "body of knowledge."

–Karen Myers

Chapter One

Affliction, Onset, and Crisis

Change is generally considered stressful. A negative change in health is of great consequence. The writing in this chapter illustrates a variety of situations. Some authors tell of the initial onset of an illness or physical condition; others tell of a crisis or an episode of reoccurrence. Each author has his or her unique reaction to the situation, but all are dealing with the unknown.

Crohn's Disease

Rachel Naomi Remen, M.D.

There are those who wake
in the same body every morning.
Ankles and knees moving briskly, unaware.
Belly, painless and unnoticed.
The breath the same,
as full, as sweet,
as when they laid down last night.

I awaken every morning and wonder
What body I am in today.
What moves freely? What aches?
How clearly will the right eye see?
The left?
What will obey? What rebel?

Uncertainty is aliveness,
and aliveness,
grace.

from Perfectly Normal: A Mother's Memoir

Marcy Sheiner

In 1956 my brand new transistor radio brought me the startling news of a pair of twins born with their heads stuck together. My ten-year-old imagination took flight, boggled by the possibilities. Did they share a brain? How would they walk? Most of all, what did they actually look like?

Excitedly, I ran home to deliver the news to my mother and my aunt, who was pregnant at the time. "Maybe," I said hopefully, "you'll have babies with their heads stuck together." My aunt gasped. My mother slapped me.

Wounded, I shut myself into my room to reflect on what I'd done wrong, but try as I might, I could come up with nothing. Apparently, these marvelous creatures I'd heard about weren't considered so marvelous by the grown-ups. It would be many years before I understood why.

* * *

August 3, 1965.

I awoke to find myself in a room with a woman sitting up in the bed next to mine, pulling metal rollers out of her long brown hair.

"Hi," she said cheerily. "My name's Jackie. God, am I

glad for some company. Now that I'm leaving tomorrow they finally bring someone in here. Isn't it always the way?"

I smiled uncertainly through a sodium pentathol induced haze.

"I had a boy, too," Jackie continued. "They'll be coming around for feeding soon. You'd better let the nurse know you're up if you want to see yours."

Without hesitation I obeyed this stranger who, by virtue of having given birth a day or two before me, qualified as an authority.

The nurse appeared in less than a minute, whirling through the room flinging open curtains, flicking imaginary specks off the sink. "Oh, so you're up, Mama," she said with a nod in my direction. "Have you urinated or had a bowel movement yet?"

I shook my head, remembering my sister Linda's vivid descriptions of the excretion ceremonies on the maternity ward; I knew if I didn't urinate they'd catherize me, an altogether unpleasant affair, and that I wouldn't be allowed to leave the hospital until I'd emptied my bowels.

I strained on the bedpan, examining my body. My belly was loose and flabby, still patterned by purple stretch marks: so, I was stuck with them for life. My vagina was a pathetic mess, having been not only assaulted by a razor, but cut and stitched as well, episiotomies being as much a routine of childbirth as cutting the umbilical cord.

"Have you done it yet?" called the nurse.

"Not yet."

"Well, dear, I'm going to have to catherize you."

Threatened with invasion, my bladder immediately

released a healthy stream of urine. When the nurse returned with her equipment, she actually seemed disappointed.

"And now are you mommies ready for your babies?" Jackie and I nodded eagerly.

My newborn son slept in a tiny glass box perched atop four wheeled legs. At first sight he resembled my grandfather, or any old man, his red face scrunched up in denial of his new surroundings. The nurse gave him to me with a bottle of water. He took a few weak sucks, then fell back asleep. Jackie's baby sucked avidly.

"Don't worry," she assured me. "Mine didn't drink the first day either."

Holding Daryl, I felt far older than my 19 years. For the first time I questioned my decision not to breast-feed—I had thought it old-fashioned, an activity suitable only for cows, an attitude enthusiastically endorsed by my family, friends, and doctor. Well, it was too late now—I'd been given pills to dry up my milk.

Surreptitiously I unfolded the blanket and took a quick inventory: ten toes, ten fingers, all in the right places. One tiny limp penis. Relieved, I closed my eyes and leaned against the pillow. Jackie's voice startled me. "Aren't you glad he's all right? I was terrified something would be wrong with my baby. But thank God, he's perfectly normal."

"Yes," I breathed, recalling the nightmares: attacks on my swollen stomach, hideous creatures clinging to my vaginal walls.

Every pregnant woman harbors the fear that something will be "wrong" with her baby—but to give voice to such thoughts during the nine months of gestation would be to give them greater credence; admitting those fears is as much a part of the afterbirth as the bloody placenta.

* * *

In the evening visitors filled our room. Jackie's husband and mother stood quietly by her bed, while my mother, father, sister and Bob, my husband, filled the rest of the space.

"Hey toots," my father boomed affectionately, giving me a wet kiss, grinning from ear to ear. When he smiled, his cheeks reddened like tiny apples in his shiny round face.

My mother pecked the air near my cheek, then took up a position at the foot of the bed. She stared without self-consciousness at Jackie's family and asked in a loud voice, "What did she have?"

"A boy too," I murmured, wishing that for once my mother would keep her voice down. But she went on, talking about the nurses, the hospital décor, her disdain of the crosses on the walls.

"It's a Catholic hospital, Ma," I said in a low warning voice.

"Yes I know," she replied, her words dripping with animosity. The only aspect of Judaism practiced in my family, so far as I'd ever been able to make out, was an active dislike of the goyim.

Bob had brought a bouquet of roses, and Linda ran off in search of a vase. When she returned she made a great fuss with them, searching for a knife to cut the stems, filling the vase, arranging them just so. This domesticity was totally out of character; I wanted my older sister to sit down and commiserate with me about the maternity ward, but she seemed to be avoiding any intimacy.

Bob's face was covered with thick stubble, rendering his dark olive skin even darker. He slouched in the corner chair next to my bed, inexplicably subdued.

My father grinned from ear to ear, and my mother sported her usual stiff smile, worn through thick and thin—but I had the uneasy sense that they were disappointed in me. Maybe it was because I'd had a boy—in my family we coveted female babies, dolls to dress up and show off.

Everything was discordant. Feeling acutely uncomfortable, I felt a sudden unstoppable urge to pee—a tedious event that involved pouring a pitcher of water over my stitched bottom in lieu of toilet paper, a procedure which everyone in the room could not avoid hearing. I should have been embarrassed, but I was too caught up in more confusing emotions, and the bathroom afforded me an escape from the claustrophobic atmosphere.

The next morning my obstetrician, a young crew-cutted fellow with an upturned nose and pasty skin, came in to check on me. As he poked at my breasts, lumpy with the strain of unreleased milk, he mumbled, "We're a little concerned about the shape of the baby's head. We're going to run some tests to see if he has hydrocephalus."

Life stopped. My heart skipped a beat; my facial muscles froze. The world narrowed, and it would never, never look the same again.

"What are you talking about? What's hydrocephalus?"

"Oh," he said casually, "it's a disease that causes the head to grow abnormally." He pulled up the sheet and headed for the door; hesitating, he groped for a comforting phrase. "Don't worry," he finally managed, "you can have more kids."

I sat there, totally stunned. So that was why everyone had behaved so oddly the night before: something was wrong with my baby. I should have known, dammit—should have known that a girl as clumsy as my mother always said I was could never pull off an uncomplicated birth.

Jackie broke the cold silence. "You're worried about what he said, aren't you?"

"Yeah. What's he talking about?"

"Oh, I wouldn't worry. It didn't sound too serious." She hid her face behind a hand mirror, and didn't speak to me again. I hardly noticed when she packed up and left the hospital with her baby, but sat immobilized, thinking not of my baby's probable pain, not of the uncertain future, but of the past: the past nine months. What had I done wrong?

I had conceived under less than ideal conditions: in the backseat of a car, unmarried. In a panic, I married a man who was a virtual stranger to me.

During my pregnancy I'd had a vaginal infection, and, having no notion of what the itching signified, felt too ashamed to tell the doctor.

I had watched my weight rather than nutrition, starving myself prior to checkups, and was proud to gain only sixteen pounds total—dieting was encouraged by my doctor, who'd asserted that "eating for two is an old wives' tale"—but now this became another one of my personal wrongdoings.

In my ninth month I'd gone swimming in a public pool, only to learn later that some doctors advised against this.

Last, but certainly not least, I had made love beyond the allotted time limit, up until three short weeks ago.

The litany never ended. With each passing day, year, decade, new sins were added to the list. Cigarettes. Coffee. Alcohol. Aspirin. I devoured reports of new medical discoveries, acquiring ammunition against myself. Sodium pentathol: I should have had natural childbirth. Radiation in cow's milk: I should have been drinking soymilk. Zinc. Calcium. Iron pills. Every time that child cried in pain or staggered under the weight of his head, my heart would cry out mea culpa.

Foggily, I climbed out of bed to join the other mothers walking up and down the corridors in their new E.J. Korvette bathrobes. I saw them as characters in a science fiction movie, machines that had fulfilled their baby-making function, now useless and bored. I don't know, maybe they were walking around in a state of grace, ecstasy even, but as I said, the world had narrowed.

Or perhaps it had widened.

* * *

I walked to the pay telephone and began dialing Bob's office, but stopped midway, remembering his demeanor the previous night: surely he had known. He had known something was wrong with our baby and he'd deliberately kept it from me. I hung up the receiver and sat in the phone booth absorbing this information.

Never had I felt so betrayed. However well-intentioned were Bob's motives in withholding vital information from me, I would never fully recover from this sense of betrayal; if we'd been strangers when we'd married, we were now well on our way to becoming enemies.

I picked up the phone again and called my sister.

"Linda? I just found out that the baby might have something called hydrocephalus."

"Dammit. Who told you?"

Again the bottom fell out of my world. "You mean you knew?"

"Well, Bob didn't want you to know until you'd had a chance to recover from the birth, so we all had to act like nothing was wrong."

My husband. My sister. My parents. I was surrounded by a band of lying traitors.

Stunned, I walked slowly back to my room. Bob was sitting in the armchair next to the bed. He didn't notice me at first, so for a minute I was able to observe him. Suddenly he seemed smaller than his six-foot-four and two hundred pounds, weaker than the burly football player he was, more vulnerable than the barroom bouncer he'd been when I'd met him. My anger at him dissolved, as I realized that he too was suffering. This baby was his child also; his first child; his son—with all the weight that word carries for a man like Bob. He looked up and, seeing me, opened his big bear arms. I fell into them, sobbing.

Silently we comforted each other. Finally I said, "To tell you the truth I can't imagine this happening to anyone else we know."

"What do you mean—you think we're losers?" he asked.

"Yeah," I said softly, feeling a great wave of shame flood over me. "That's what I mean."

I had, after all, failed the greatest test of womanhood—for women ultimately prove their worth by bearing healthy children. Indeed, in the recovery room Bob had whispered, "You came through with flying colors, kid." Now I'd learned that I had not, in fact, delivered flawlessly.

I had not been a rockbed of self-esteem to begin with; now I felt as if some inner deformity had manifested itself in my child, who would henceforth provide living proof of my defectiveness.

The hospital suspended normal visitation rules, allowing Bob to stay with me all day. On and off I cried, on and off I raged. I wanted the baby to live. I wanted the baby to die. I wanted the baby not to have this disease with the evil-sounding name.

When Daryl was brought in for feeding again, I studied him with a more critical eye. I saw what I'd missed before: his head was only slightly larger than normal, but asymmetrical. Tentatively I touched it: it seemed so vulnerable, he was so vulnerable. I felt a fierce desire to protect him, and at the same time, a certain amount of fear—not fear of what might happen to him, but an inexplicable fear of him, of his strangeness.

My parents came to visit again; this time we had the room to ourselves. My mother stood at the foot of the bed, smiling brightly, chattering inanely.

"We're getting the room ready," she said. No preparations had been made before I went into labor, out of the traditional Jewish superstition that this might hex the outcome of the pregnancy. Thinking of this archaic ritual and how it so obviously meant nothing, I laughed bitterly and said, "Ma, you do know about the baby, don't you?"

"Know what?"

"About the hydrocephalus."

"Oh, that. So, he'll have an operation."

Her characteristic lack of emotion suddenly enraged me. "You don't care, do you?" I shouted. "You don't even care!"

Her smile never wavered, but her eyes burned like dry ice, imparting their usual message: Get control of yourself.

I had no intention of getting control of myself: my mother had known something was wrong with my baby, and had marched in here smiling. Worse, she had somehow led me to this hospital bed with never a hint at what might transpire. A husband might betray, a father, even a sister—but a mother was not supposed to betray.

"You're like some kind of robot," I shouted, sobbing hysterically. The nurse, who must've heard the commotion, came scurrying in.

"Visiting hours are over," she announced briskly, shooing everyone out, though there were at least another fifteen minutes left. After she'd emptied the room, she returned with my usual vitamin pill and, beside it, a new pink capsule.

"What's this?" I asked.

"Just a little something to help you sleep."

Dutifully, I swallowed my "medicine" and awoke the next morning not only refreshed but optimistic. Suddenly I, like my mother, felt that nothing was terribly wrong. When I thought about it, what was the big deal, after all? My baby had a medical problem; the doctors would fix it; and we would all live happily ever after.

The pediatrician came to explain my baby's condition and probable operation. Hydrocephalus, he told me, is a disease of the central nervous system wherein cerebrospinal fluid, rather than circulating normally, accumulates in the head, causing it to grow rapidly and exerting pressure on the brain. The word literally translates as "water on the brain," a phrase commonly used to denote stupidity in popular "jokes," a phrase that would from this day forward cause me to cringe reflexively. In the past, I learned, babies with hydrocephalus either outgrew the condition—sometimes with brain damage—or died. In the late 1950s an operation was devised wherein a plastic tube, or shunt, is inserted beneath the scalp, stretching into the chest or stomach cavity, draining the fluid. Daryl's head was only slightly larger than a normal infant's, so his prognosis was good.

Under the effect of pills, which I never suspected until years later were mood elevators, I began to view Daryl's condition as if it were no more significant than a mole or a wart.

When my obstetrician came in later, he asked if the pediatrician had been to see me.

"Oh sure," I said, waving my arm in the air. "He told me all about hydrocephalus. Did you know Winston Churchill had it and he outgrew it?"

"No, I didn't," said my doctor, frowning as he checked my breasts.

"Well, he did. But I guess Daryl's going to need an operation."

"Hm. Well, anyhow, you can have more kids."

I snapped my gum in his face, mentally willing him out of my consciousness. "Daryl is going to be fine," I said, despising him.

My grandfather called to suggest institutionalizing the baby.

"Just think," he reasoned, "you'll be stuck for the rest of your life."

"He's going to be fine, Grampa," I said. I rolled my eyes at Bob, who was trying to follow the conversation, and mouthed something about my senile, old grandfather. "He just needs an operation."

A friend who'd heard something was "wrong" with my baby telephoned.

"Oh," I said casually in response to the concern in Louann's voice, "he has something called hydrocephalus. They're going to do an operation and then he'll be okay."

"Thank God," she said. I could almost hear the rosary beads clicking in her devout Catholic hands. "At least it isn't a missing limb or something really bad."

"Oh, no, nothing like that. Really. He'll be fine."

Bob was astounded by my change in attitude. Beneath my bravado and drug-induced oblivion, though, I was feeling more and more isolated from the mainstream of humanity, a feeling that would intensify and affect me for the rest of my life. There were those who, like my grandfather, acted as if Daryl's birth was a dire tragedy, while others, like Louann, were relieved that he didn't have "something really bad." Both attitudes denied reality. Neither left room for my complex bundle of feelings . . . For who could ever understand the depth of my disappointment?

I may have gotten pregnant by default, but the truth was, I had wanted a baby for as long as I could remember. I adored my little cousins, and once I was respectably married, I'd been ecstatic to be pregnant—in fact, I'd admitted guiltily to Linda that I had, at least subconsciously, engineered my pregnancy. I basked in the doting smiles of strangers as my belly grew, and devoured books on child rearing. I fantasized dressing up my baby, taking her (invariably I imagined a her) out in the stroller, playing with dolls in our apartment. I couldn't wait to have my very own little baby, for in my limited experience, babies were delightful playthings.

Most parents eventually learn that babies are much more complicated than mere playthings. I learned it in one brutal day.

The Joy of Polio

Pierre Delattre

I jumped out of bed on a morning of my seventh year and fell flat on my face. There was no feeling in my legs. I managed to pull myself onto the bed while screaming for my mother. She got me laid out on my back, then hurried to get my father. He ordered me to stand. I tried but once more fell. He put me in bed, propped me up on pillows, raised an eyebrow, asked a few questions. When he learned that I would miss final exams if I wasn't in school that day, he demanded to know what kind of game I was playing. Did I think it was this easy to get out of taking exams? "Stand on your feet!" I said I couldn't, I just couldn't. "He's faking," he told my mother, and walked out. Now I wept not only at what had happened to my legs, but at my father's disbelief. I'd always made straight A's, I argued. Why would I want to skip exams? She hurried downstairs. I heard an argument. Then my father was standing over my bed again. "Do you know what somebody has when they can't stand? Polio! Yes! If you can't walk, then you have polio. Infantile paralysis! Shall we have the doctor come fit you with braces? Maybe put you in an iron lung? Or would you prefer to get up now and go to school?" He had to be off to work, he said, because life was no joking matter, and he better not find me in this bed when he came home. Understood? My mother took my temperature, saw with dismay that I had no fever. "Grandma's going to keep an eye on you. I have to go substitute teach. I can't play this game any longer. If you're still in this bed when I come home, I'm calling Dr. Bailess, do you hear? House calls cost money. Think of your embarrassment if he finds out you're perfectly fine. Think of the spanking your father's going to give you tonight." "I'm not faking!" I screamed with such anguish that my mother stepped back, stunned. I saw her struggle with doubt. "We'll see," she said. She left me. I tried several times during the day to get up, but my legs remained useless. I had polio, I told my grandmother. I knew I did. I finally convinced her. She phoned my mother at the school. Around five, Mom arrived with Dr. Bailess. He examined me, took her downstairs, murmured something. I heard her body thud to the floor. I listened eagerly. When she had recovered from her faint, I heard their slow climb up the stairs. They entered the room. He was helping her stand. He gave me a friendly smile. She looked at me imploringly through her red-rimmed eyes. He told me there was every reason to believe that I had only a mild case of polio. A few weeks in bed with my legs propped up on pillows, who knows, I could be walking again. "Really?" I said. "I have polio?" Oh, how happy I was. I had polio. I really did. I couldn't wait for Dad to get home. I'd show him! *

---

*I want to thank my brother Roland for dragging me to my feet day after day and insisting that I try to walk. Without his persistent encouragement and faith that I could, I might not have recovered.

Another Asthma Night

Dustin Michael

Relax . . . find it . . . turn on the lamp. Find the inhaler—the knife that cuts the snake off my throat. Find it . . . FIND IT . . . before the brain realizes it's suffocating. It always thinks the strangest things while dying, desperate attempts of a panicked intellect trying to distract itself. It never helps.

Where is it? Why isn't it under the pillowcase? Rip up the mattress, quick! Throw it down! Shake the blankets! Relax . . . relax . . . breathe . . . focus . . . breathe . . . find the inhaler, cut the snake off. Pockets! Check the jacket, the jeans. Where is it? Pillowcase! Maybe it's inside the pillowcase; maybe I shoved it inside there before bed, instead of underneath. Feel inside the pillowcase. Relax . . . breathe . . . focus . . . focus . . . it feels like drowning . . .

Drowning, yes. She was underwater so long and there I was, clinging onto that tree in the river with the upside-down canoe bobbing methodically, spilling out our camp gear and zip-lock bags of lunchmeat into parts unknown downstream. She was down there, under the tree, kicking for her life in the submerged brambles, and all I did was stare downstream and scream and scream. "Chrissy!"

Our stuff was all over the river and it was quiet except for that song in my head—*Closing Time.* It was on the radio every 10 minutes that summer. "I know who I want to take me home" played over and over, and she was still underwater, and all the while I was screaming "Chrissy!" and it dissolved right off my lips. *I know who I want to take me home, take me home.* "Chrissy" isn't a name that grabs hold of the wind and rides, like "Jesus" or "Mommy."

Focus . . . breathe in! . . . find it . . . breathe out! . . . in the backpack . . . in! . . . zipper pocket . . . out! . . .

Mommy? Mommy—she wished her kid would never take for granted a single breath. And just look! See your shining son now, Mommy? He's an all-grown-up big boy with a big boy apartment, and just look at all his big boy things everywhere! Nobody says, "Clean your room! Vacuum and dust your room!" now. Nobody shouts and takes away his big boy things, like Mommy did with his teddy bear when he wheezed. There's no Mommy here saying, "Big boys don't need dusty old teddy bears, just their big boy knives to cut the mean snakes off their throats so the Mommies can sleep. Where's your big boy knife, Pumpkin?"

I know who I . . . in! . . . *want to take me home* . . . out! . . . *I know who I* . . . in! . . . *want to* . . .

There were mean snakes in the brambles where she was still underwater kicking and drowning, and they were hissing "Chrissy!" like a wheeze in the lungs of the wilderness where the teddy bears go after the Mommies take them away at *closing time, you don't have to go home but you can't stay here* . . .

Here! . . . in the grocery bag . . . why in the grocery bag?? . . . hurry . . . cut the snake . . . in! I'm OK. I'm OK. Relax. Breathe. God, why did I put it in the grocery bag? It's so late. Work tomorrow is gonna be hell. The mattress is leaning up on the wall like a crippled soldier. It's late. Get blankets, get pillow. Go sleep on the sofa, or try.

That song's gonna stay jammed in my head for weeks.

I should call Mom tomorrow. And Chrissy. I found her down there in the tangles, and I pulled her out. She was fine. We went out for another year and a half after that trip.

Jesus, the mind thinks up stupid things when it's dying, but who knows? Maybe she's still underwater. Or maybe it's me.

Red on Blue

Donna Kichner

It happened again. It happened so unexpectedly. Now I'm on the floor—and it isn't because someone has asked me to dance. Oh, my God. I'm bleeding. I focus in on colors. Bright red blood is splattered all over the pale blue carpet. I place my left hand behind my head to find that my hair is soaked. What should I do now?

I look all around me to see if there is a phone nearby. There it is—about twelve feet away on the divider between the couches. I've dragged myself that distance by my elbows on several previous occasions. But there are differences this time around.

My mind begins to wander. It latches onto the first occasion of seeing red on blue. I was fifty years old and had already suffered several strokes. I was still walking unassisted and was just about ready to leave home for work. I had forgotten to pick up my counted cross-stitch project that I wanted to have with me. In scurrying back to the bedroom, my right foot brushed too closely against the carpet and I fell against the doorjamb. A small amount of blood splattered the carpeting. That time, however, I was strong enough to pick myself up using my left hand. I was able to regain my balance, walk to the nearest phone, and call for help. This time, things aren't so easily done.

My mind focuses on another occasion similar to

my present predicament. I was on my way up the cellar steps, when I decided to stop and change the cat litter. The unexpected weight of the litter box caught me off balance and I tumbled backwards. By that time, I relied on a MAFO brace to strengthen my right leg and a hemi walker to maintain my balance. I pondered what to do, because I had no phone within reach. As the damp, cold cellar floor pressed against my skin, I summoned up enough strength to get my body upstairs. I dragged myself to the base of the steps using my elbows for support, picked myself up using my left leg and my left arm, and managed to hoist myself up the stairs and onto a chair at the dining room table. Success. I made a quick call to a neighbor, who helped me stand upright and handed me my glasses and my hemi walker. Everything was under control again. But that was then, and this is now.

This time, the knit fabric of my sweatsuit creates friction against the carpeted floor. This time, my head is bleeding and I have no way to be sure of the extent of the wound. I decide to get as comfortable as possible and wait until my husband returns. He is only about two miles away, working on the rain spout of the nearby post office. I have learned to be patient on occasions like this—and to make use of the waiting time by thinking and singing. No tears or self-pity.

I check my watch for the time. It's 3:15 p.m. For a while, I lie flat on my back with my left arm cradled behind my head. When I sit up fifteen minutes later, I notice a fresh patch of blood on the carpet. Something tells me I should confine myself to a seated position, and so I try to relax in the center of the living room floor. I glance around once again to be certain there is no furniture I can use to pull myself up to a standing position. I succumb to just waiting for help to arrive.

Three hours pass. Finally, my husband comes home. He hoists me up using my armpits as a leverage point. Then he hands me the hemi walker and asks me what happened. I tell him that I bent over to dust the entertainment center, lost my balance, and fell backwards against the hard oak magazine stand.

While he gets the carpet cleaner out to work on the bloodstain, I prepare myself for another trip to the hospital emergency room. My slacks have to be changed since I wet myself during the long wait. I manage to clean myself up and look quite presentable. About two hours later, with seven staples implanted in my skull, I emerge as good as new.

from Falling

Clint Pearson, M.D.

Blood squirts from my thigh, and I drop the syringe to clasp it tight.

"Ursh, come quick! I must have hit a vessel."

I feel fire climbing up my body to my face. It carries hot bile to the back of my throat, but I swallow it back down. I shake my head to remove the bad taste. Ursh is here. How'd she get here without coming through the door? Who cares? She's panicked, and her mouth is open, making noise. I wave her away. I just can't deal with her problems right now. Oh, shit, the fire's trying to come out the other end. I scramble to the toilet and make it, barely.

I must stink, but the fire's burning my nose and eyes now. It's in my throat again, making me burp. I wave at the shower. Ursh understands, turns it on. Bless you, Ursh. I'll handle your problems after the shower, after the fire's out. I promise.

Ursh is helping me up. I hope she doesn't breathe. I must stink. Ursh's face is squished like a bruised peach. I must stink bad.

I'm in the shower now, water's cold, feels good, and the fire's no longer on my face. I swallow some water. I need to get the water inside but it doesn't work. The outside's cold but the inside's hot, way too hot. My body's burning inside, everywhere, flaming, flaring. I must have swallowed firewater. Typical city water. It's not worth it, too much chlorine. Damn the water bill, I won't pay it.

The fire's still burning. What's the matter with our water? It can't seem to get in. How do I get it in? My legs are burning inside. Close the door Ursh, you'll get water on the floor. I need all the water to put out the fire. It doesn't help me on the floor. Why is she looking at me like that? Just let me take a shower. Can't a guy take a shower these days?

I'm just tired. That's it, just tired. Why am I standing? I need to save my energy. It takes a lot of energy to fight a fire. I'm moving down, slowly, slow-motion drama like the six-million-dollar man. I'm tired, I need to rest, to sleep. The shower's making a lot of noise, pounding and screaming. Turn it off, Ursh, turn it off, please. The water stops. I'm psychic. Or is it Ursh? It's quiet, except for the dripping. Too hard, though. Tomorrow I need to remember, remember, remember, to put a pillow in the shower.

Wouldn't you know it? Here comes the fire again. Can't run, no sense in it, just fan the flames. Forget it. I don't want more water, too loud. What does Ursh want now? Fuck it. I can't deal with any of it now. She doesn't make sense. Blah, blah, blah, blah. Who cares? Fuck it, I'm going to sleep. I'll help Ursh with her problems in the morning. Tomorrow . . . in the morning . . . wait . . . no no no . . . deal with it then . . . in the morning . . .

"Clint. Clint. Can you hear me?"

Jeff, what are you doing here? I'm trying to sleep, but the floor's too hard. I got to remember to put a pillow in here. Remember, remember, pillow, pillow.

"I'm going to pull you out."

All I need's a pillow, but since you're already pulling . . . Man, watch the rail, that's rough on my butt . . . Now that's soft, very soft but still no pillow. Oh well . . .

Damn, this is a bad idea. The carpet's way hotter than the shower. Here comes the fire again. Maybe, if I'm really still and go to sleep, it won't see me. Still, still, don't breathe. Crap, too late, I'm burning up. I need ice, ice water. No! No! I need back in the shower. Oh shit, it's too far. I can't make it, can't breathe. The fire must be stealing my air. I need air now, fast. "Call 9-1-1." Fast, fast.

Lights red when eyes close and breathing hot. Fire in my mouth in my belly bubbling out flowing fizz-slow thick like lava but my eyes shut see red just red see fire are fire now. Now floor is fire fire floor lapping trickling burning on my back neck face eyes throat furnace-hot boiling blowing. Loud blasts boom turbines screaming screeching into my ears my head deep down flushing full sizzle. Drop and roll, drop and roll. Let it go, go go go, just let it go be still be still just find it find something good soothing good water. Bumblebee sting-hurt stuck sticky legs on arm but buzz buzz buzz, buzz away, buzz away gone now. Now floor rocking rising floating above flames into dark cool-wind shiver quiet . . . fluttering away from fire choke and humming softly space empty. Just sleep now just sleep . . . sleep . . .

Lights, fluorescent and moving like railroad tracks, whisking by, but place is active, familiar. What train am I on?

"Trauma room two."

I thought I finished my shift at the hospital. What's on my arm?

"What's the story?"

"33-year-old male, Dr. Pearson, presents with nausea, diarrhea, and fever of 105.9 after injecting some multiple sclerosis medicine called Copotone—"

"Copaxone. It's called Copaxone, and I'm burning up." Man, these lights are bright, and everybody's crowded around. I can't fucking breathe.

"Dr. Pearson, how are you feeling?"

"Very hot. Gotta get this fever down–fast. I–can't–handle–fevers–this–high–can't breathe."

"First, just tell me what happened."

"No, Ramirez, no time to talk. Pack me in ice." I feel cotton-dry drool tumbling from my mouth but can't move to wipe, can only spit it out with my words.

"It's alright. You injected your medicine and then—"

"No! No time! Pack me in ice!" My eyes burn my sight crimson, and I cough out what feels like dusty cobwebs, only they're hot.

"It's alright. We'll get your fever down. Amy, get him 600 milligrams of Motrin. Any allergies?"

"No, no, no. I can't take fever this high. Pack me in ice, damn it!"

"Just relax. It's alright."

"I am not delirious! Pack me in ice or get the fuck out of here!" My face is flaming. I see Ursh, and she looks like she did when her dad died. Now she's looking at me like I'm crazy, but I know, I know. "Pack me in ice! Pack me in ice!" I scream-spit the words to Edie, a nurse, who blinks and glances at Dr. Ramirez. He grimaces, mumbles, and walks away.

Amy enters as he leaves. "Here's the Motrin."

I swallow the pill, but it's difficult; I choke. My throat

is dead, seared and disconnected, slowly filling with dry, airy spit. I have to keep coughing, spitting, just to breathe. I'm losing my airway, drowning in heat and these people want to talk blah blah blah. Fuck you! "Pack me in ice, pack me in ice now."

Everyone's looking at me as if I just yelled to rip out my eyes and cut off my penis. Wake up! Wake up, it's me, and I know, I know. "Pack me in ice!" The two nurses, Amy and Edie, freeze, blink wide eyes at me, and look toward the doorway.

Suddenly, I see Jeff. "Jeff, Jeff, get them to pack me in ice."

He looks at his shoes and stammers like Jimmy Stewart in *It's a Wonderful Life*, "Well well, I-I-I'm not actually working you know."

"Then I'm working, damn it. Pack me in ice!" Jeff shrugs and looks like he just swallowed something bad, expired milk, perhaps. Edie leaves, and I look at the ceiling for a moment but have to turn back, panting, gagging, hoping that the ice is on its way.

Ursh touches my face with trembling fingers. "Ursh, are they getting ice?"

"I don't know, I don't know." Her voice cracks like fine china held too tight.

Edie returns but only carrying an ear thermometer.

"Okay, let's see where we're at." I can't feel the thermometer, but I know it's in because I hear the beeps. "105.4—you're hot."

"Edie, pack me in ice. Pack me in ice now!" More froth spills onto my chin and seems to bubble around my mouth, but I don't care as long as I can still breathe. "Pack me in ice before you have to intubate me." Somebody give the fucking order.

Edie looks at Jeff who shrugs, and then she hurries out the door, quick and quiet, like a burglar, and returns a moment later with clear-plastic bags of ice.

"Open the bags. Tear them open. Put ice on my crotch, under my arms, and then go get more." I don't feel the ice much—cool like a spring breeze, perhaps, but definitely not cold.

I'm calm now, directing the ice burial, watching serene and surreal as my body vanishes beneath the glassy chunks. The others are grinning, chuckling and shaking their heads, smirking tightlipped and glancing about, as if they were children stealing chocolate cake and finger-painting it on the kitchen counter. I breathe slowly in and out and shake my head, smiling. Ursh smiles too.

In a few minutes, I feel the change, unseen and soundless, void of even a shiver, but as distinct as a candle in a cave.

"Okay, start to pull some of the ice away, slowly, no rush. Leave the ice under my arms and on my belly and my groin but take away the ice on my legs and arms."

"Are you doing better?" Ursh looks unsure, probably apprehensive that I will demand the ice be returned.

"Yeah, I'm cooling. I'll be fine in a little bit. Ice is a wonderful invention."

"Okay, Doctor Iceman, let's check your temp." A little cautiously, Edie approaches, as she would an intoxicated patient. The thermometer feels hard and cool this time.

"Better, 102.1"

I wipe my mouth with my right hand. It's a little clumsy, feels like a piece of wood, but I can move. The wood thuds back to my side, crunching and shifting some ice.

"I don't think I'm ready to do micro-neurosurgery, but I'm better, and, maybe, tonight I can do my wife if she's not too hot."

"I'm way, way too hot for you, Mr. Ice. I'll melt you." Ursh grins, and her face relaxes, but her eyes refuse to leave me, even as the others laugh.

Five more minutes and my body shivers a little.

"Okay, help me remove the rest of the ice and then I'll sit up."

"You're not going anywhere. Dr. Streeter is on his way so just sit tight." Edie looks confident now, like she's through with taking orders from a patient, but she does use a towel to remove the remaining ice.

"Clint, don't be a pain, not now. You need to wait. And don't give me any of that invincible stuff." Ursh uses her best stern face to cover a slight grin.

"Relax, I'm not going anywhere. I just want to sit up to stretch my lower back."

With Jeff on one side and Ursh on the other and my legs still dead, I raise up stiff and straight bending at the waist, like a vampire in a coffin. I know I can't stand yet, but a smirky idea strolls into my mind.

"One thing's for sure, we need to contact McNeil Pharmaceuticals right away."

"McNeil? Why? Do they make Copaxone?"

"No, they make Motrin. I'm sure it was the Motrin that cooled me down so fast and saved me. We need to buy some stock."

At first, Ursh just stares, squinting and scowling a little, her mouth half-open, trying to find the logic, but I can't hide my smile forever, and she soon sees.

"Oh, would you just get serious for once in your

life?" Ursh tosses ice at me, and her lips pout out her smile, sly and smoldering. "Next time you better listen to me. None of this would have happened if you had just listened to me. Next time I think I'll just leave you in the shower. How would you like that?"

"That's alright, as long as you get naked and join me, baby, or, at least, bring me a pillow."

Chapter Two

Isolation, Preoccupation, and Recovery

We can become isolated from others all too easily. Sometimes a flare-up prevents us from doing what we had planned, or pain forces us to withdraw and detach—even if we struggle against it. We may need to act in ways that are not understood. Often, those around us don't know what to say or do, and we may feel alienated. The writing in this chapter examines how living with a physical condition can separate us from others.

Migraine

Ryan G. Van Cleave

Only a few minutes more for the pain pills to work,
I watch the September rain steadily glaze the windows.

I feel dizzy-drunk without the pleasure of having had a beer
or vodka on the rocks. The water beads on the glass spin

with reflected streetlamp light. I know the pills confuse me
and my head is speared with hot needles of headache,

but those waterdrops are tears. They're coming out of
the window; the glass is crying. I reach out to touch it

but stop short, not wanting to disturb the bizarre display
of sorrow. What would a window have to be sad about,

I wonder, but my muddled head refuses to uncover an answer.
There's a lightning flash and the eventual thunder echo

is a twisting sound so unnatural and drawn-out I know the
pills are putting me to sleep. But I know what I know.

There are tears on that window. Anybody could see that,
pain pills or not.

from

Glowing in the Dark

Barbara Lehmann

Barbara has discovered the power of her presence. Who cares if her family doesn't know what to say to her at the dinner table? After all, dinner table talk can be trivial. Please pass the potatoes and thank you very much will do quite nicely. Just to be there is enough to belong. That's it, that's the key: she's going to have to start making her own rules here. And rule number one is that no one gets to imagine what it might be like after she's dead. Because no one is checking out early here.

Feeling invulnerable, she decides to check in with Coco before she goes down to dinner. Coco can't hurt her any more than she already has. In fact, a real confrontation with her friend would provide the perfect opportunity to display her newfound strength and humanity. And to tell the truth, she would just like to chat.

"Hi, Coco!" Barbara wonders if Coco even realizes how she hurt her feelings by not being there for her.

"Hey, Barbara." Coco sounds as impervious as ever.

"What's happening?"

"Not too much."

"Me either." Be brave, she reminds herself. Say what you mean. And yet, she can't bring herself to form the words: I miss you.

Coco suddenly sounds sheepish. "I was going to call you."

"Yeah? I guess I beat you to it." That's good, Barbara bolsters herself. Keep it light.

"Last night was the Boat Dance."

"That's right! I forgot," she lies.

"It was fab."

"It was a beautiful evening last night."

"It was perfect. You should have been there."

"I know. Wish I was." Don't sound pathetic, needy. "I had a hot date with the TV. I saw this old movie, *The Diary of Anne Frank*, a real tear-jerker."

"You shouldn't watch things like that."

"Why not?" Barbara swallows. The movie actually came awfully close to portraying exactly how she feels, cooped up in the house. "So. Don't you want to tell me about the dance?"

"Sure."

"I count on you, Coco," she appeals to her friend.

"I wish I could tell you in person."

"Hey, why don't you come over after dinner?"

"Can't. Got a paper due tomorrow. I haven't even started yet. You wouldn't believe how much homework they give," sighs Coco. "You're lucky to be out of it."

"No, I'm not." The truth.

Silence.

"Didn't Mark tell you all about the dance?" Coco hedges.

"My brother was there?" What a shocker.

"Yeah, he came with Tasha. You didn't know?"

No, the creep. "I know they're in love."

"I'll say! I saw them making out pretty hot and heavy on the deck."

"Big deal. I've seen them touching with their clothes off!"

"You have not!"

"Have too. So tell me about the dance."

"There was a real crowd. They rented a cruise boat from the Red and White Fleet."

"Huh," Barbara grunts. "So, how was your date?"

Silence. Is Coco trying to keep a secret?

Then she blurts out, "Oh, Barbara, he's simply the grooviest guy I've ever known."

"Wow." Barbara hadn't expected that strong a response.

"He's a perfect gentleman, opening doors for me, helping me on and off with my coat. He's a great dancer—and a great kisser!"

"Coco!"

"It was the best evening of my entire life, totally romantic. When the band took a break, they put on *Sergeant Pepper* over the speakers, and you know that's my favorite record, and then Jim and I when out on the deck. That's when I saw Mark and Tasha."

"Oh."

"It was a real scene. First we just watched everybody else going at it and I kept thinking, ohmigod, I know we're going to do it, too." She starts giggling.

"Did you?" Barbara can't keep the agitation out of her voice but Coco doesn't notice.

"Yes." More giggles. "First we went to the edge of the deck and looked at the moon's reflection rippling in the current. It was so beautiful, and then I felt his arm creeping around my shoulder."

"Creep sounds like the operative word of that sentence," Barbara throws in, but the sarcasm is lost on Coco, who is immersed in the blissful narrative of reliving last night's events.

"And then he turned me to him or maybe I made the first move, I don't remember exactly. His face was so close and his lips were closer and then he pressed them against mine. Oh! It was great! The first kisses were kind of hard and awkward and then we just melted. His lips got all soft and warm like mashed potatoes and . . ." Her voice dwindles in ecstatic memory.

"Did he put his tongue in your mouth?" Grossness is tempered by a ruffled edge of excitement.

"Yes."

"Ohmigod!" Barbara squirms at the thought. It should have been her.

"And that's not all."

"What do you mean?"

"I can't tell you."

"You have to." The taste of experience is too tantalizing in her mouth.

"Well, we were making out for ages. And he was so tender and gentle and loving," Coco purrs.

"And?" She can feel herself get hot with anticipation. If only she'd been there with her own boyfriend.

"And I was so excited I could have jumped into the water. And then I felt his hand on my back and I couldn't believe it. I mean, his fingers were on my bare skin! Somehow he had unzipped my dress without my even knowing it. I mean, I don't how or when he did it. His hands were really warm. He has the strongest, roundest arms of anyone. I think he's going out for football next year."

"Good grief, Coco, and then what?" Coco's commentary is driving her crazy. If only she would stick to the event.

"Well," Coco continues, "He was kissing my lips and my cheeks and my hair and then he started kissing my ear and I just went crazy. I mean, you can't imagine what that feels like."

"Oh, I bet I could." Pleasure so sweet it is painful.

"It was unbelievable. Like he was blowing right into my love center. I don't know where he learned to kiss like that."

"What else?" She tries to keep the envy out of her voice.

"Well, one of his hands was on my back and the other was traveling around me like . . ." Her voice breaks.

"Like what? Did you let him feel you up?" She scratches at some non-existent itch on the back of her neck.

"Yes!"

"Ohmigod! Coco!" She is impressed. The only person who's ever touched her breasts is a doctor. "Over or under?"

"Both. I mean, there was just no stopping his hands. Before I knew what was happening, he must have unhooked my bra."

"You're joking!" Barbara wipes invisible sweat from her forehead.

"I'm not. And I thought, I can't let him do this. The nerve of him! He'll lose all respect for me, but like, I couldn't tell him to stop. I didn't want him to stop. It felt so good."

A vast heartache burns in her chest. Barbara gulps breath as if it could put out the fire.

"So, I let him touch me on my breasts for a while."

"I can't believe it." Barbara grabs a handful of hair and holds tight as if to anchor her own libido.

"Me either. First I was so shocked, I was sure he must think I'm a stupid slut."

"Did he say anything?" Barbara reflexively checks her hair for split ends. "No. We didn't really need to talk. It was so romantic. I really love him." She pauses to reflect upon her love.

Barbara is speechless.

"I don't know," Coco sighs. "After a while, I guess he kinda fixed my bra and zipped my dress and then we went back in and danced some more."

"Wow."

"I know, I can't believe I'm telling you this. I feel like a dumb whore, but I'd do it again in a minute. I just can't wait to see him again."

"When's that?" She combs her fingers over her head to keep cool.

"He called me this morning. He told me it was the best dance he'd ever been to. Me too, I told him, me too. I'm in total love. This is it. I'd marry him tomorrow."

"Well, you don't have to go that far." Lifting her hand to her face, she is suddenly holding a handful of unattached hair. She stares at the hunk of strands in her hand.

"I know. He's coming over later and we're going to talk."

How many hairs is she holding? One hundred, two hundred? She shrieks in horror.

"What?" Coco sounds guilty. Barbara blanks out for a second. Suddenly, she realizes she's got to get off the phone. What were they talking about? "Didn't you say you had a paper due tomorrow?"

"I do," Coco misunderstands, caught in her lie. "But I can't do anything until I see him again. I can't think of anything but him. Jim Conner. Isn't that the coolest name? Coco Conner. It's perfect."

"Coco Conner?" Barbara repeats in disbelief. This isn't happening. She runs her fingers up her neck and through the bottom of her hair. Another handful comes out.

Coco's tone flips from fervor to fury. "Well, who asked you? I think it's super. I'm so happy I could just die."

Die? Barbara has stopped breathing. She pulls another lock of hair from her head. It comes out all too easily. Something underneath her skin just next to her skull is pushing follicles right out of her scalp. It's as if her head has lost its glue and can no longer keep the roots in place. Her head is spinning. She gasps for air saying, "Maybe you guys could commit double suicide."

"Shut up, Barbara, you're so mean. I was afraid of that. I didn't want to tell you anything. You're just jealous."

"Right. I'm just jealous." Can't talk about it. Can't stay on the phone. Her eyes smart. A white mass of fury forms in her guts and bounces into her eyeballs. She feels dizzy. Rage and panic. Got to get away. "I have to get off the phone." Whose voice is that? She sounds rational. "You have to get ready for your date."

"It's not a date. We're going to talk."

The last thing Barbara wants to do is talk. She wants to scream and yell and kill people. "I have to go." Go where? There's no escape.

"Don't be mad, Barbara. You should be happy for me."

"I am. But I gotta go. Bye." She hangs up quickly. As she stares at the three handfuls of hair lying in her lap, tears stream from her eyes, blurring her vision, and she can no longer focus. The horrific facts stare her right in the face. Her hair is falling out just like they said it would.

It takes every ounce of strength in her body to make herself stand up and walk into her room. Hair in hand, she goes straight into the bathroom and locks the door. She looks in the mirror. A mass of hair is scattered all over the pink sweater her mother brought back from Italy last summer. The hair shafts, having simply let go of her scalp, have fallen into a bed of clinging pastel mohair. A forest of trees, become suddenly rootless, has started to wander the landscape. Her hair has left her head.

Pulling a strand of hair from her sweater, she thinks, "This is happiness. Throw it away." Another one, "This is joy. Goodbye." She adds the strands to the mass of hair already gathered. "This is love. This is faith." She will have to find a pretty box to store them in. A coffin in which to bury hope.

Falling to her knees, in front of the mirror, she just wants to sink to the tile floor and die. It's too painful to look out from behind her eyes. Her eyes, so like her mother's, her father's, her sister's, her brother's. The family resemblance so striking, with characteristic dark hair. Her hair. Thoughts so bleak, she can't stand them any longer. Pressing her face close up to the glass, she surrenders to the darkness. Closing her eyes, she kisses her own lips in the mirror. Its surface is cold, unyielding. This is it, she realizes. This is goodbye. "It's all over for you, my darling."

Sick

Merry Speece

When I close my eyes, a pink angora sweater in a landfill, a creepy thought.

I've been lying here a long time. In this bed where I have, through the years, turned adversity to my pajamas. Every morning when I wake, I ask, what will a new day bring? A newspaper. Besides *that.* No, just a newspaper.

So in the early hours I lie in bed longing for the day's newspaper. My energy reserves in thimblefuls, I hoist one up and rise for the news. At the front door's the paper, and in the sky my moon's still there. Moon, when are you ever going to help?

I step back from the door, the morning, and the world. My hip joint gives. So, it's one of *those* days, when a leg doesn't want to stay in the socket.

Back to bed. Now:

Housed. Laid down inside.
Sharpening stone in dull water.
Or–No. 0 biscuit in its slot.

I take up the paper. The sentences of the newspaper swim, the news washes over me. Other people's lives. Humanity.

Lay it down, all too much, to rest.

And now for the Poetry Minute, about all we can stand.

Timepiece
Look at the little clock that's been
Fucked to death.
Wind-up watch, pocket watch, body heat.
In the desert, I am Dali's, not upright.

If only I could get a message to Emily Dickinson through that messenger boy God. That's what I do as I lie in bed. Think of my pretend friends. Right into the future I chase Cesar Vallejo trying to make him wear a condom.

Welcome
Death
the boy unrolls the long white condom for me

When the phone rings, it is, as I figured, my daily wrong number. People try, day after day, to reach Human Services. I'm glad enough to hear a human voice, and yet how anxious and baffled and ashamed the poor sound caught trying to go on relief. If it weren't for the grudging support of next of kin, I could be one of those calls myself, and I could dial wrong just as easily as anyone and get my own busy signal.

I used to have a beau, and he called. That was so long ago, however, I can hardly remember. It was another life.

And yet—I still love him. And I might be able to say just how much if only I had that *Software Classic* MATH RABBIT.

Your promise to me was
the Krispy Kreme Promise.
I could always count on you
for freshness.

To him I used to write the most passionate letters. But I gave up writing when I couldn't do it, too much in love, without getting that telltale sore throat on the right side.

Double my grief
Like a wedding
like Death the Bride

I feel as if
once I held a sack
of grain
and spilled the seed
and we both sagged down

Love for me in the millefiori.

To be honest, a man did call for me—what was it?—two weeks ago? Woke me from a dream. It was the loveliest dream of my beloved kissing my fingertips and opening my palms to his lips and then down the insides of my wrists and on to the tender skin of my forearms.

On the phone was the heat pump repairman, Elbert "Pee Wee" Sweat (real name, as it appears on his card), and shortly Pee Wee stood at my door, come over at last to add freon. "You put that stuff on your hands, and your hands'll drop off," he said, proffering the tank—threatening. Then when I walked out to show him where the unit is, and I leaned close to the machine, he growled, "Keep your fingers away from there, or you'll git your fingers cut off."

When he'd called, finally, to respond to the pleas I'd left on his answering machine, I'd heard this strange voice say, "This is Elbert Sweat. Remember me?" though I'd never met the man. *Remember me?*—the question in a bad dream and *your fingers'll git cut off, your hands'll fall off.*

This makes me think of a dream I had the other night. The key to the dream was a German word, but when I woke up I couldn't quite remember and struggled for the right translation. The place in the dream—what was it called? The place, no it wasn't Liebestraum, Love's Dream

on the summit of the wooded hill this castle
no monastery no now that my time has come and
I am inside and see nuns we are obliged to call
it what it is convent

Lebensraum in the history of cruelty some people
have become a cliché these nuns just as bad I
am a prisoner in the Leben the Leben something
and either this is the 90s or I am in my
nineties I am old and on the shelf with
yellowed scrolls one of which is mine that a nun
will draw out to read the expiration date on the
day she and the others will facilitate my death

I must escape my old bones ache my aching bones
the pain thank God for the tunnel Pain this
way the quickest exit out of Lebenstraum

In another dream I was looking for a grave marker. I mean I was shopping for one and trying to see what I could get for the fifty dollars in my pocket, all I had. The one I found was slight and brass and competently bent 'round rather in the shape of a music stand. The grave marker was for my own grave.

Let the music begin.

An alarm! I am reminded of the world out there. Someone's security's gone off.

No, crazy, that's a chickadee, the way chickadees *insist.* God, and sometime last week the sound of a cricket I mistook for a disk drive going bad.

The weeks go by, long, like eels, and unelectric.

I'm bored to death, and I may get up in a moment and turn on the lava lamp to watch. At last night's viewing, the lava flowed up in a staircase to the top. When the heat rose, and the stair collapsed, at the bottom was revealed a one-armed person with their head against the glass. Apples fell and piled around the poor thing. The apples rotted or melted and lost their shape, and then yellow fluid bubbled up under the red lava, and red balloons rose and blistered in the liquid sky, and the blisters broke, and the red balloons shuddered, redder and more perfect, and continued to rise. Down below, the person collapsed in the heat, lava pouring from pelvis or big leg stump.

Other times I lie on my back and look up at the reflection in the globe of the floor lamp that leans in over my bed. I meditate on the life of The Girl in the Globe of the Gooseneck Lamp.

She lies there in the white iron bed that curves around her. A door and two windows, a bookcase and many books, lean. She's the center of a cell, sealed off, waiting for a miracle.

Waiting, more like it, to meet her Maker on the Day of Poor Judgment.

Her mouth is small in sorrow. Eyes recessed in dark hollows smolder. Her face could hardly be rounder.

Her head is big, her feet, so far away, barely there. When she reaches out, the arm that appeared normal at her side, fattens, bruises swell, the ragged patch of rash erupts, and here's a hand huge in your face.

It's one of those days when she feels as if the flesh is coming off the bones of her forearms. Her bones sing Klingon opera, aria of warrior's torture. She's short of breath and coughs.

She made the mistake yesterday of trying to escape into the world. And in the middle of the night she woke with shirt drenched. Later intense itching on her back and fingertips disturbed sleep again. At dawn when she came to, both little fingers and both little toes had lost feeling.

Now she tries to collect her thoughts through pressure in her head.

She lies there and what does she worry about, how terrible it would be if an asteroid hit Serpent Mound.

She lies there and daydreams about living in a little house on a bend in the road and feeling each traveler take her curve slow.

She writes in her head: I am as leaden as a Roman General. Gone down. In armor. Under horse hooves. *Landslide.*

Sometimes she cries a little.

Chernobyl, we are sick.

And what, you ask, you foolish person, what about a miracle?

Thusly, said the magician.

Myself in the Stone

Josh Danoff

Last night I felt the weight of stone on my spine as I slept. Felt bolts of pain travel up from my knees, spiral around my waist, and stop at the small of my back. The pain sat there and rested, waited and grew round and dense like a concrete ball, and lodged itself where my spine curves in a little too much.

In the morning, I open my eyes and reach for my knees. I feel them breathe, beat quick, short pulses around the bottoms of the kneecaps and up the outsides. I touch them and they are warm. I clamp my teeth together, close my eyes, and exhale the pain, pretending to feel nothing. I stretch my legs out until the knees lock, and then bring them back in. I hear things going on, moving around underneath the caps. I feel the clicking, feel the grinding and scraping of cartilage and bone meeting. Something is very not right, I think, and swallow some water.

I feel like drinking sometimes and wish the doctors would let me so maybe the pain could have somewhere to go. But they say no, because of all the antibiotics, because of the nature of Lyme disease. My primary care physician won't prescribe the medication I need for the pain, so I take lots of the ones he will.

Later, when I am driving, his nurse calls me back on my cell phone. "I'm just the messenger," she says. "You should make another appointment to see a different orthopedic surgeon if you don't like what the other one had to say."

I pull the car over to the side of the road. "I already told you that I did, with McBride, but it's not for three weeks. What should I do until then? I've tried everything I can and have been waiting a real long time now to see somebody."

"Oh good. You're lucky you got an appointment so soon; he's supposed to be very good. The doctor said he'd write you a script for Naproxin."

"That's an anti-inflammatory, right?"

"Yes."

"I've used that one before and told you I can't take it because it hurts my stomach too much. What about oxycodone maybe, or something like that?"

"He doesn't feel comfortable prescribing you that."

"I don't feel comfortable in all this pain."

"I'm just telling you what the doctor said, Josh. I can't make him change his mind."

I want her to tell the doctor that I think this is bullshit, that the majority of my experiences with him and his office have felt like a goddamn battle. I want him to know about the miserable receptionist who makes me feel like I've done something horribly wrong just by calling. He should also know that I've wished terrible things on him, that I'm not a violent person, but if given the chance, I'd love to take his inability to listen and his incompetence and beat them into him. I'd laugh at him there on the ground, helpless now on the other side of his medicine, and walk away.

Instead I sigh and say, "Fine. Yeah, okay." I hang up

and know this is not one of those times to get angry or yell at the voice on the other end of the line. I'm too tired, I guess, don't have the energy for it anymore. I just say, "Fine," and punch the roof of my car when the nurse hangs up. I turn the radio on and rock my head up and down to the music. I close my eyes and run my hands over my face.

Maybe I'll go get some coffee. Fuck. I drive into town and park, hop out of the car, and tuck my head deep inside the fur hood of my jacket. It's February and the ground is covered with snow. I walk into the bakery and ask for a slice of cranberry bread and some coffee. The girl behind the register recognizes me and we exchange smiles. The bread is warm in my hand and I sit down and rub my knees, pushing down in certain places with the hope of finding somewhere they won't hurt so much, or maybe even go unnoticed.

I take my jacket and drape it over a chair. Steam rises up off the coffee as I place the lid on a napkin; it spirals into the air and disappears. I bring the cup to my mouth and am not so cold anymore. I look around at the other people, warmer now too, and watch their lips move, make up the words I'd hear if I was there on the couch with them, or sitting in the chair across the table. How I'd nod and smile and respond with words of my own.

I look out the window; it's too cold to snow today. The wind shakes the bare branches of the trees that line the road and whips around thin sheets of old snow. I see a woman walking into the wind, wearing a long black jacket, a pink scarf, and a matching pink hat. I see her face taste the cold, and as she exhales, her breath is a cloud for a moment before she gets flustered by the wind blowing away her scarf. She shakes it in the air and looks around, then wraps it snug around her neck.

I look away from the woman and back into my coffee. I know what I'll say to the nurse the next time I call: "Do you not believe that my knees actually hurt? Think maybe I'm just saying all this to get narcotics? Think I want to be all fucked up, lying there in bed staring at the television, having my brain numb up so I can't think straight or talk right? I don't want all that. I just need to do something about the pain."

It is May of last year when my symptoms begin. The air outside is heavy and thick. I can smell the hot, feel it in my throat, feel the stick on my skin as the heat latches on. I wake up at night scared and breathing hard—the outline of my body drenched into the sheets. My temperature swells to 103 degrees, and the doctors take blood and guesses. During the next three months I tell them about the pain in my abdomen, how it moves up my left arm to my neck and shoulders, and finally to my head.

I believe the doctors when they tell me what the tests show, what they don't. They give me pills that are supposed to make me better, and I don't question them. I think that because they speak in this exotic language filled with big, strange, important-sounding words, they must know what they are doing, know what is best for me. They are professionals.

Instead, the pills make me worse, sicker, until one night in July I try to take a sip of water, but it spills out of my mouth and onto my shirt. The doctors call it Bell's palsy. They say there's a swelling in my brain that has pushed up against a nerve causing me to lose control of the left side of my face. I go to the emergency room and they put all the symptoms together. They take more blood, this time to test for Lyme disease, and spinal fluid, to see if it contains white blood cells—which would mean meningitis. They find the cells they don't want to and are sure the Lyme test will come back positive in a few days.

I lie on a stiff mattress with crisp white sheets and a pillow that is neither hard nor soft, but some strange place between. I watch the ceiling and see the lights whiz by over my eyes. I hear the tuk tuk tuk of the stretcher's wheels clicking over slits in the floor. There are big, round mirrors attached to the corners of walls where hallways intersect. The edges of everything look soft in the mirror, but distorted too, especially when I get a glimpse of myself rolling down the polished hospital floor. A woman wearing light-blue clothes wheels me to a room for overnight guests of the hospital. The room has two empty beds and she puts me in the one near the window.

"Light hurts my eyes," I say, and although it is night, she shuts the blinds.

She touches my shoulder and wants to know about the pain. She says she'll be back in a minute and returns with a syringe. I feel cold liquid travel quickly up my forearm—the muscles tense and harden as it seeps out of the vein and seems to expand in my arm, pushing the skin to the point where it might explode if everything continues as it is. Then nothing. The liquid hits the bloodstream and instantly moves throughout my body. My arm deflates. I lean far back into the bed and feel my chest slowly moving up and down. I listen to myself inhale, then exhale, as my eyes slide from side to side, as the lids open and then snap shut.

My hands stay flat next to my body, or maybe resting on my chest, either way, too heavy to lift. Yet they seem to move somehow, feel like they're floating up above the bed and drifting around in front of my face as my body slowly, steadily rises and falls with an imaginary tide. There is a tingling, a numbness about my whole body. The pain inside my head—the piercing grind of sharp points that seems to start inside my eyeballs and work its way around to the back of my scalp—seems to subside, dull for a moment.

Later, I look around but no one else is there. If I can find the button that makes the head of the bed move, I can press another one and a nurse will come in. During certain parts of the day and night, I have to press the button a few times and wait before someone asks if I want water or juice or if I am hungry. I try to figure out if I am, and what I'd do with the food or water once I got it. I tell them there is pain, bad pain, and half smile when they come back with a syringe full of morphine. I'll try to sleep now, or at least close my eyes. I'll lie still and breathe, dream away the pain, let my eyelids slide down and all my muscles go limp. I leave the television on the news so I can hear sounds other than hospital noise. Tomorrow people will come to visit and say things to me; I hope I'll be able to understand them and respond with words of my own.

The morning after I leave the hospital, a nurse comes over to my apartment and delivers the antibiotics that are to be administered daily through a pump. "Remember," she says, "with that line in your arm you can't do any physical labor—you can't lift anything over ten pounds."

She shows me how to sterilize and attach the tube at the end of my arm to the pump. The tube connects to a line that runs up my arm to my shoulder, and then around toward my heart.

"Ten pounds, shit. How will I be able to work?"

"You won't. You're sick. You need the rest. Isn't there any paperwork you can do for your business?"

"Yeah, but not that much. If I don't work, I don't make money."

"Sorry," she shrugs, "No work."

After six weeks in bed, I finally go to the job site. My nurses are appalled, but I need to keep an eye on the helper when my business partner isn't there. Then I start going even when he is around. It's hard to be there—sometimes harder than lying in bed—just standing around watching the guys work, straining their bodies lifting stones, seeing the veins turning purple and blue and raising up off their arms.

I stand with my arms folded or resting on my waist, anxiously shifting my weight back and forth from one leg to the other. I pick up a shovel one day and work for fifteen minutes, then go home and lie in bed for six hours. Twenty pounds underweight, I feel weak standing in the unfinished driveway surrounded by piles of stone and trap-rock, helpless and unable to lift rocks, even drive the truck or operate the Bobcat. I shuffle my feet in the dirt and watch the minutes tick by, trying to think of ways to waste time.

I think about my health and in which direction it is moving, where it might go next. Time enables everything to be gone over and gone over again. Picked apart and scrutinized, examined like medical charts and the tiny drops of blood that get placed on thin rectangular pieces of glass and slid under microscopes.

I stand in the yard and watch—watch and wait and want to work, but know I can't. Unable to lift my arms and carry my own weight, I wish my body to work like it once did, will my hands to pick up tools and wield them again like I used to. I shake my head and close my eyes.

I reach into the tool bag and know again what it's like to work with stone. The way the rubber grip of the mason's hammer gets sticky with sweat and slips around inside my hand until my palm is hard, until the folds of skin on my fingers where the knuckles meet are calloused. I exhale and feel my forearms constrict, feel the power and weight of the hammer as it strikes the stone and crumbles it, as rock folds under its solid metal head, and bits and pieces of stone fly up into my face and chest. I like to see the silvery dust from the rocks coat my hands and arms and clothes; it acts as a measurement of my time, tells me I'm doing something.

I feel sweat dripping down from my forehead into my eyes and mouth, and search for a clean piece of shirt to wipe away the salty liquid. My arms are slick with moisture. I feel like a man again, strong and powerful as I crush stone with the hammer and it splinters. Country music plays in the background and I half-consciously sing along. I smile as the rock sheds layers of itself and grimace as I pick it up, as it tears the skin and digs into my stomach—its shifting weight balanced gingerly on my knees, buried deep inside the small of my back. I smile again as the stone slides onto the wall and into place, snug against the one before it and neatly cradled by the ones in the course below. I step back and study it, making sure the joints are tight and clean. The wall looks good.

And like nothing, I'm back. Instantly in the groove again, picking up stones and hardly having to touch them with the hammer because I already know that they'll fit into the wall just right. Look guys, I'm back, like I never left. Easy as pie. I open my mouth and yell out as I heave a rock off the pile in order to expose the one I need to keep building. I'm moving faster now, and faster, my arms and hands and eyes and body working together on their own. Like riding a bike, yeah, a bike—just hop on and go, start moving. No matter how long feet haven't touched pedals, they still know what to do; they don't forget. I look at my hands and feel the hardened skin, and know they remember, too, remember everything.

I open my eyes and look down. I'm wearing sneakers on the job site and my hands are soft and clean. My tools lie in their bag and there is no silvery dust on my clothes. I look around at the piles of rubble littering the driveway and see the wall being constructed. I see the piece of Styrofoam on the inside of my left elbow and the plastic tube that runs to my fingers. I see a small bit of string that signals the beginning of the pick-line. My arm hurts and I start sweating. I get inside the car and find the bottle of painkillers. I throw a few in my mouth, close my eyes, lean the seat as far back as it will go, and wait.

Today, I look out my bedroom window and see the backyard covered with snow. I want to know where the warm has gone, where my time has gone. I want to miss staying up late and sleeping in. Want to rise with the cold, with the dark, and work until the dark at the other side of the day comes. I want to lift stone again, have it become lighter and lighter as I move faster, floating around to the different piles, and having the rock seem to rise off the ground, up into my arms as we carry each other to the wall and become a part of something. Something alive and tangible. Real. Real as the hands that shape and sculpt the stone, real as the sun that burns down and turns my neck red, drips beads of sweat down from my forehead into my eyes and mouth, and real as the day that starts and ends in the place between light and dark. I want to see myself in the stone, in my work. Stone does not lift itself, shape or build alone, but I am not there now to help it along the way, nor for it to help me.

Pap Goes the Wheezer

Sharon Wachsler

Recently I went to the local feminist health clinic for my annual gynecological exam. Nobody enjoys these visits, but if you're a woman with a disability they can feel like you've landed an appearance on the freak-of-the-week show: just when you think it can't get more humiliating and outlandish, you find yourself sitting on the damp pavement in a dark parking lot actually hoping that soon you'll be inside the clinic—a stranger peering into your nether regions, yanking out pubic hair as she wrestles the speculum into place. But that comes later.

The day starts deceptively smoothly. My friend Heidi picks me up in plenty of time to navigate the dense Boston traffic. Heidi is taking me to my appointment because I have multiple chemical sensitivity (MCS). I get ill when exposed to small amounts of common chemicals, such as those in perfume and cleaners. I know that by the time I leave the clinic I will be too sick to drive.

Our first mistake is that we arrive at 4:00 p.m. for my 4:00 p.m. appointment. Heidi goes ahead to give the receptionist my name. "The doctor is expected back by 4:30," the receptionist brightly informs us. She is wearing a colorful blouse. It looks like several tropical birds have landed on her chest.

"Where is the doctor?" I ask.

"In another building," the receptionist answers, startled. I am arrayed in a stunning ensemble of assistive equipment: a carbon filter mask (white, it goes with anything), an air filter on a cord around my neck (classic black, always in style), and an oxygen tank (basic metallic green, on wheels, for that "gal-on-the-go" look). I don't think she expected the mound of technology to speak.

Because the brand-new clinic reception area reeks of perfume and various other chemicals, Heidi and I decide to wait outside. "Always avoid vomiting in the reception area" is one of my cherished rules of etiquette.

We wait the extra half hour in the parking lot. For an hour and a half. Cars and trucks idle nearby while harried drivers search for parking spaces; buses grunt out diesel fumes on the corner. Cigarette-smoking, cologne-spritzed Berklee School of Music students saunter past us, making me wish I could wait somewhere else, like an oxygen tent.

It gets dark. It gets cold. We sit on the ground, trying to avoid the cigarette butts. Finally a nurse comes out to give me a form. "Since it's dark and your fingers are numb and your brain has turned the consistency of nonfat yogurt, we'd like you to fill out this illegible form" is what I imagine her saying. What she really says is, "This form may be a little hard to read in places." She is right. One of the places it is hard to read is the parking lot.

Here is a copy of the form, from what I could make out:

Medical history: afdndfj stupojj quentosnwabbi?
Yes/No (Choose one.)

Check one: past, present, outpatient, impatient, future imperfect, subjunctive.

Check all that apply: heart, lungs, gastrointestine, thyroid, an-droid, gastropod.

Check one: sibling, parent, grandparent, grandiloquence, gramophone, 56th Annual Grammy Awards.

The nurse returns for the form, trailing fragrance, and leans in to talk to me. I move away, wheezing and coughing, in an effort to prevent an asthma attack. Heidi explains to the nurse that I'm reacting to a scent she's wearing. The nurse snaps, "I'm not wearing anything!" This makes me feel much better.

Finally we go into the examination room to wait for the doctor, whom I really like. She's gentle and caring and laughs at my jokes and generally treats me like a human being, which I find fun and refreshing, like a cold drink on a hot day—with a little umbrella in it—maybe something orange and fizzy that comes in a neat "upside-down" shaped glass like you would get on a Caribbean island where you lounge on the beach, a papaya-scented breeze blowing through your hair, music playing in the background, maybe something by Miami Sound Machine, and the band leader looks over at you, smiling, and says, "So, you're here for a pap smear?"

"Oh," I say to my doctor, who's just walked into the examination room and is looking at me expectantly, "Yes."

There is a momentary pause while she notices that I am using oxygen, which I wasn't when she saw me last year.

"Oh, Sharon!" she exclaims in alarm, "What happened?!"

I should be used to this reaction by now, but I am not. I know my doctor is genuinely concerned, but I wish my appearance didn't inspire horror. I toy with the idea of dying, just for dramatic effect, but instead explain that the oxygen lowers the severity of my reactions to toxins.

Then my doctor (we'll call her Dr. Unnervingly Long Fingernails), as she does every year, asks me various "routine questions" about my health to which I must give answers that imply that I am either a) dying (I am not) or b) a hypochondriac (I am not) or c) other (which I definitely am).

We have the exact same conversation as we had last year. Patients find routine soothing.

Dr. ULF: Do you ever have nausea, vomiting, diarrhea, constipation, blood in the stools, stomach ache?

Me: Yes.

Dr. ULF: Errr (looking at my chart, making a note).

Dr. ULF: Do you ever have painful urination, irritated urinary tract, burning and itching, frequent urination?

Me: Yes.

Dr. ULF: Do you ever have a sense of physician-induced déjà vu?

Me: Yes.

Dr. ULF: Do you ever have a sense of physician-induced déjà vu?

Me: (sighing) Yes.

The alarming nature of my responses raises the specter of extensive urinary tests or, even worse, a lubricant-dripping metal instrument the size of a "high end" kitchen appliance stuck up my butt. (You can only experience that so many times before the novelty wears off). I assure her these tests are unnecessary; the symptoms she's listed are part of my chronic illness. Dr. ULF gives me a brief lecture about how I shouldn't assume everything is related to my disabilities, helpfully suggests I may have colon cancer, and then drops the subject altogether. "Always lie to your physician" is the hint she is passing on to me.

Now that the medical history is discussed and ignored, we return to the matter at hand. Her hand.

After various Specialized Medical Instruments (speculums, swabs, fingers with the aforementioned spatula-like nails, small Chevrolet automobiles) are stuck in various orifices (cervix, vulva, Volvo) the exam is over, and Heidi and I return to the reception area to pay. We are fortunate that Heidi is with me because otherwise the receptionist would have no one to talk to when she speaks to me. Apparently, based on my using assistive equipment, the receptionist decides that I am not able to converse with her and refers all her questions to Heidi. This is true even when I have answered her previous question.

Our Actual Conversation:

Me: Can I pay here?

Receptionist: (to Heidi) Does she have a co-pay?

Heidi: (pointing at me) I dunno.

Me: Yes, it's five dollars.

Receptionist: (still looking at Heidi)

Heidi: (finally) Yes, I guess it's five dollars.

Me: (tearing out the check and putting it on the counter in front of the receptionist) Here.

Receptionist: Will she be paying now?

Heidi: (pointing to my check on the counter)

Receptionist: (staring with vague expectation at Heidi)

Me: (picking up the check and waving it in front of the receptionist's nose)

Receptionist: (taken aback) Oh.

Nothing beats the thrill of surviving an annual gynecological exam and pap smear! I'm ready to celebrate by going to bed for several days. But, truly, I try to remember that, despite the fact that they worsen my medical condition, annual exams save lives—not to mention, they pay for my clinic's new reception area.

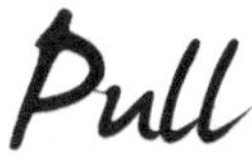

N.M. Moro

I never chewed on my braids. I pulled them, twisted each strand of ebony brown. My mother never told me to stop. I believed it was OK.

One's hair is one's crown. It determines one's character, distinguishes the "mussed" from the "put together." I have never known how to put myself together. I have always pulled.

I pull and twirl my bangs, twist the short hairs until they are shorter, miniscule, gone. I was blessed with a crown of thick, strong hairs. I have made them weak.

It's the awareness that kills me. Being fully aware that I am stuck on something toddlers do. That even if I shaved my head, I'd find a way.

A self-help book tells me to postpone obsessing. There is no putting off my pulling. Yes, I claim it as my own, as a part of me, so intrinsic, so strong, it has been with me since birth. If I could will my hand away I might, but I might not. Failure to pull is betrayal, not giving in is danger. Pulling brings me to safety, protects me from what is and what might be. It is often the only thing I can be sure of.

There are pills for these things, but so far they haven't worked. They have aggravated the urges. My urges get angry, too. Angry when I fail to satisfy them. Angry when I don't comply. They tell me I have failed.

Losing hair, losing mind, losing touch. I'm prematurely balding, my scalp red and patchy from the pulling. And the sound. The sound of satisfaction, breaking, breaking free. It's a comforting sound. I hear it in my sleep.

I can't separate obsessions from compulsions. Pulling is both my obsession and my compulsion, something sacred, reserved for the searing times of anxiety and angst, times on the edge of safety and madness. My hair is thin, like the fading line between crazy and sane. I don't know which I am. And so I pull.

Recovering Darden

Caitlin M. Warde

I've got about fourteen Starbursts in my mouth. The place under my ears is tight, trying to keep up. He always tells me that I eat white-trash candy. He wonders why I never touched his Baby-Ruths and why I can't stand him touching me.

The phone rings and it's someone I don't know. My mouth is full and I attempt a "he's not here right now."

Sitting at the window, I trace lint off the pane. The garage view, he would say, is, after gross inspection, unremarkable. I disagree. My silver Jetta is thin, has lost its gloss in the wind, its flanks ulcerated with uneven rust rings. The car shudders in the filth of the garage, and I imagine the crackle of gasoline fumes, sweet in my nostrils.

My insides are jumping and I hear his voice leaving hours earlier, saying take it slow, let it heal. And ever since, I've been here, in the recliner, slouching on the brink of action.

I imagine the Getting Better. It is slow, like a diagnosis. It took them eight months to name it: Crohn's disease. Not colitis, or anorexia, or irritable bowel. Richard agrees with them, that my hair will make a Great Return. My arms are still sore from the poking. My abdomen weeps brown, thick tears that burn when I move. I cannot wear pants. I cannot eat corn or lettuce or his Baby-Ruths.

He's somewhere near. In the anatomy lab again, I'm sure. Carving up Tropical Carl, his own personal cadaver. I saw him once peeling off its skin, dark and wet. Carl's face (we don't really know his name, of course) is huge. His nose is heavy and ridged with the settling of cartilage. His head is shaved and I've seen his lungs. And the hair on his toes. But his hands have already been dismantled and I don't think I should go back again.

I'm not pregnant. I had been worrying though, before the surgery. Richard told me that they took out at least three feet, not including the colon. That the ulcers were spectacular. That my lymph nodes all had granulomas. That I was this close to having a perforation. That I was lucky he made me talk to a surgeon. That I was lucky I lived so close to the hospital.

The pain is bad. He'll tell me why. He will name each knife of musculature. I quiet myself with some Coke and a couple of Percocet.

The phone rings again and the machine clicks, his "hello-this-is-Richard-and-Darden" and the rest. I listen and wait. My brother wants to know what I'm getting Mom for her birthday. He's thinking a new toaster oven, or maybe I should buy her a sweater and put his name on the card. He assumes my proximity to a would-be pathologist fills my bank account. He hopes that I am feeling better. My brother and sister are fraternal twins and don't look a thing like each other. This has always baffled our mother. Two eggs, I told her since the fifth grade. I have offered to diagram it.

When I met Richard he was all "hi-baby-whaddarya-drinkin'?" I told him a pearl diver and he was all "that's cool," and he got me another. I was healthy then, and he was in his second year, just done with genetics, aced the exam, invited to do a research project, and I let him tell me all about fraternal twins, my eyes open to the brow. I got stuck in the rough corners of his face, the way his voice curled around my name. That night, I let him sleep with me.

Tacy was supposed to call. She hasn't and the dog won't let me touch her. The super-chew rawhide was a mistake, I guess. She has cornered herself with the slimy orange barbecue stick. I can smell it from the chair and it makes me queasy.

Tacy was Stacy but she went through a Dark Phase, Richard calls it. She wore all black clothes and pierced her ear with a third hole and dropped the S.

Tacy smells like old closets. She wears men's wing-tip thrift store shoes that curl up at the ends like witches' hooves. When she talks, her voice stays mostly in her throat. That fleshy resonance makes her seem deep. She has dark patches on her face that look like iodine splashes. She always tells me that she has olive skin.

She began to fade once I got sick. She said that she would call when I got out, though. Richard doesn't like her. He says she's a crackpot. He says she should have visited me in the hospital. That she's been my best friend since junior high. I don't like to think about it too much. I wish she would call.

I want to watch soap operas but the remote is out of reach. I can't force any more pain on myself. Any movement hurts. Maggie is no company. Now her tongue and teeth are completely orange. She leaves a mark on my leg with her licking and leaves the room.

I want to make a list, precise with dates and times and names. I want to recognize myself again, my arms, my calves, my face. I look like a snowman, my rounded segments barely together, my eyes like raisins, dark and hidden in the swell.

I would like to get lost in Greensboro again, driving fast as the quick triangles of pine flash by. I would wind for hours in the loops of Wendover Avenue, avoiding the concrete canals of highway that devour landscape, that have digested beauty. All of a sudden I want to swim at the beach, or trip like I did in high school with Tacy, or buy a new recliner.

I miss going to the grocery store. I would stop at a Winn-Dixie and gather raisins and Watergate salad and those pre-made burger patties for Richard. I won't eat meat anymore. Ever since he described Carl's aorta I just can't.

Carl didn't die of a heart attack, though. It was prostate cancer. It's a funny thing, that prostate business. Quite honestly I don't know where it is. Down Low. Down There. All of Richard's oncology friends are always saying not to treat it. It grows so slow usually that they die of something else first. My Carl wasn't so lucky.

I think about how cold it is in the basement of that hospital. I remember the recovery room, how I woke up too early, how I surprised the nurses with my sudden demand for drugs. The doctors, with their spidery faces, all men. I told them to stop lying. I told them to give me something: their Morphine, their Valium, Versed, a placebo.

A nurse in surgical colors told me she' d fix it. That I should stay still and stop calling out for Richard. That they're not doing anything because I'm hysterical, I'm a woman. She directed a small black man to my table to put needles into my spine. He was blocking it, he said. I concentrated on his voice, the parts that stayed above water.

I think about Richard now, the little hairs on his neck. And I wonder if he is with Carl.

I want it to rain or snow or to heave something definite from the sky, something dramatic. I want to reach up and feel it, to have the clouds brush through my arms, their salty residue between my fingers. The horizon meets the cement outside in a single heave of blankness. Its weak light seeps through the pane. The anemic rays cough through sporadic clouds, their thin hue expiring in my palms.

I whistle for the dog, longing for her to collapse against me. I want her warmth. There is no response and I hope she is okay.

I look at the shoebox on my desk, crammed full of medicine. Almost a month ago the dog ate some Cyclosporin and Prilosec. I rushed her to the vet and they pumped out her stomach. Her stomach, no bigger than my fist, spasmed as she cried on the cold table. Richard's still mad about the four hundred dollars.

Richard again lingers with me here. I think of his sighing in his labored sleep. He tumbles through each REM cycle, waking me with the blinking mumble. His movement strangely comforts me, my still limbs balancing the mattress. When I ask him, he says that he loves me, the way I even us out. He loves me for our symmetry.

I can still smell Richard. It won't wash off, the smell of chemical preserves like honey and formaldehyde. The smell of Carl's flesh. Richard swears he wears gloves in the lab, but I know he doesn't. Those same flat hands, the probing fingers, the analytical tips, evaluate me in the dark. I used to sleep facing him.

I smile when I think of that night we met. I can hear Tacy's "you can't be serious" jabbing through to me in the smoky noise. I sought him out with the insistent flicker of glances. I ordered that bright green drink and then he was with me. With me ever since.

Tacy isn't calling. When I try to think objectively about Tacy I remember the thin dark hair, bald in places underneath. Her arms are short. Every day, she lifts auto parts that she borrowed from her father's garage. She tells me that she wanted to feel a muscle somewhere. She chose there, above the rough elbows.

It has been a while since I have heard from her. Here in the recliner, I wonder how attached she is to me. I long for her joking and our joint candy consumption. I think about our trips to restaurants (me paying) and how she always brought a book for herself for the times I had to run to the toilet. After a few minutes she would check on me. Sometimes I cried afterward in her car and she said "oh baby, oh" and held my head on her lap.

We would drive to get lost. And once, before Richard, we drove and stayed in Asheville. Those mountain roads made me nervous. She would stop the car on a precarious turn and ignore my pleas to keep on driving. Once, she got out and leaned over the guard-rail and spit out her bright-green apple gum. When she got back in, she laughed as we speculated where the gum had landed.

I think, even now, as I stick to the warm seams in the recliner, that the gum is still there where it fell, in some unlikely crevice in the rock below. That was the best of Tacy, the way I try not to think of her.

My stomach skin itches beneath the plastic stretches of tape. Richard changes the dressing every night, after my shower. My back flat to the bed, the mattress his examining table. The reading lamp arches over my belly as he peels it back, always left-to-right. Just like reading he says. He cleans the wound, and is angered if I twitch with pain. He's not used to a living specimen.

He bends over me, his neck in the same unnatural angle as the light. His glasses sometimes slip a little and I look at his nose, wide and flared at its tip. I used to slide down that nose into his mouth. His lips flecked with my kissing, those tender rims bent towards me, towards me then.

He bandages it; his upholstery is always tight and flawless. The thick, white square is edged in adhesive. It's stiff against me. I want to tear it off and make him do it again. But instead he slips his hand beneath my back. He lifts as he gathers the tape, the gauze, and the disinfectant. They are put away every night before he snaps off the light, before he sleeps, before he places his body parallel to mine.

The drive outside is blanched, pressured numb and bloodless from the years of heavy cars. It is in even, square sections, and I can count eight of them from where I sit. There is tar spackled between each quadrangle, dark and thick and permanent. I think about the men who must have built the driveway. I wonder if they went home blistered and smelling of heavy exhaust. Did their women mind the smell of work on their hands? Did they leave a raw odor, that smell a foul echo in the morning?

My gut begins its hurting again. I can feel their hands inside, pulling dark stretches of me out.

I think of Richard, how he must have examined each ulcer in the lab, pushing his finger through until it yielded and burst with dark blood. His hands were inside me.

Richard said they felt grainy, that each circle's depth felt like sand around his finger. "Darden," he said, "Darden, you really were sick." And then he said Carl lost his hair, too. "Carl," he told me, "Carl must have suffered."

I think of Carl again, and wonder if his wife held him, cried with him. I think they had children. Three or maybe four. Richard doesn't want my children. He told me once after too many drinks that my gene pool is polluted. Polluted with my flat feet and my Crohn's disease.

They are all within me, here beneath the scar. My children, their halves huddled against each ovary wall. Sometimes I can smell the soft rotting of their membranes, each poisoned daily with the medication.

In the hospital, when the Valium finally started to stick, I wanted pearls as big as fists and a diamond for each knuckle. I swore that I would eat sugar out of my hands, its grains a sticky talc between my fingers. I laughed in little circles, dainty spirals from my throat. They came at me again, the interns, with their IV needles, with their Lidocaine sweetly burning the tops of my feet. I zoned myself to the pillow, the stitched boundary of the sheet. Each inch of me below the neck was forfeited and exposed.

They were swearing, gripping my ankle with fierce concentration. I wondered if my unshaven legs factored in, if my toenails were too long. One of them said, "The blood's got to be in there," and he jerked a smile, jabbed a chuckle. I know them all by their first names, Richard's

Sunday beer friends. The ones who would drink the Coors I bought on special.

Richard has secreted me away down here next to the phone and its machine, next to a pile of *People* and his *New England Journal*, next to wine and the bag of candy. "No roughage for two months. We taper the medicine slowly. Remember, No Guarantees." The surgeon's words are his words, tight beneath my ears. Just like the Starbursts.

The Jetta outside is peppered with old splashes of dirt. Pepper. Pepper is a naturally occurring carcinogen, Richard says. No pepper on the table or in the cabinets. None for mashed potatoes and none for me now.

I'm new. They've scooped me out clean and stitched me closed. Not even a warranty. It will begin again with nausea and groans in six months or ten years. I wonder whose bedroom I'll sleep in then, whose hands will slip beneath my back, whose calves my feet will warm between. And the dog, will she ever come when I whistle?

On cue Maggie enters, her head high, the chew's edges awkward in her mouth. She circles twice and settles next to the recliner, next to me. She is as long as my arm, feathered in grey and black. The hair on her ventral side is short, having been shaved recently at the vet's.

She's really like a cat, independent and crafty. She can jump higher than my waist and can chew through anything. Yesterday, she chewed through the toothpaste pump and ate all of the Aquafresh. Now, when she gets close I can smell that minty thickness. Spearmint barbecue.

My mind is slow, full of chemical deposits. Supposed flecks of aluminum from all the years of deodorant before Richard, radiation from all of the x-rays and scans, and thirty-four medicines that have set up camp between synapses. I know all by name. The anti-inflammatories, the anti-diarrheals, the anti-nauseals, the anti-spasmodics, and the anti-depressants. The pills and capsules and injections and inserts. They all remain within.

The body is a million lies and wrongs.

The body has an unremarkable back except for the arthritic vertebrae, those tender nubs down low. In the knee nook the blues shed the yellow. The breasts even themselves out, each as big as two fists. A veldt between the legs. The hips are white with marks the width of thumbs. Down the middle a man-made scar steals the umbilical hole.

There is no Tylenol in the shoebox and I don't think I will go up to the kitchen to get it. The pain fingers its way from the meeting of the frontal lobes and back, squeezing down through the medulla. I know each worm of brain, having quizzed Richard again and again, pushing at his scalp, naming each locale, each phrenological zone.

The recliner is brown and is torn in places underneath. Its color seems to change within the hours he isn't here. Right now it is the color of chocolate scabs, the dark flaking near the edges of a healing wound. And sometimes it melts, matching the hue of Richard's eyes. His eyes, beneath those uneven brows, their dark precision, their radial symmetry.

Carl's eyes, Richard told me, are the same color as mine. My eyes, before the surgery, were red and sore, mapped with conjunctivitis. Textbook symptom, Richard said as he pressed the lids back, his palms clamped to my cheek. After the examination he washed his hands. He was tired. He was still wearing his tie. He slanted towards me, searching through the bloat. "Darden," he said, "Darden, it's just got to come out." And for a moment he was almost holding me, his hands on my back, on my breast, on my stomach. The pain flashed from my corners and he jerked away.

He's away from me now, down in that cold basement lab. These past weeks it's been Carl's endocrine system, found and noted and labeled. I can imagine Richard labeling me, the little pins marking strange ducts, the distortions of disease.

He should also want to label the eyes, their inflamed capillaries, their reddened rims. And my fingers, each knuckle swollen, the nail beds tight, splitting the cuticle sore. The arthritic column of spine might be especially noteworthy. Those back joints swollen and pressing hard through the skin to the chair. All of me recorded. All of me to remember, the important parts counted and numbered.

Chapter Three

Reflection, Interpretation, and Spirituality

Illness often leads us into unknown territory as our familiar way of life is called into question. We may start asking larger questions about ourselves and how we fit into the big picture. The writing in this chapter explores various paths of self-reflection and spirituality: meditating, connecting with nature, recognizing synchronicities, and questioning our faith or lack thereof.

A Tough Nut

Lawrence Bradby

OK then, try to crack the meaning out of this;
Or don't.
You're right, why bother?
Why keep scratching at a sore?
It won't help find the itching's cause
And scratching will never be a cure.
So see the nurse, GP, specialist,
Then work through the Alternatives—
Starting with the cheapest, maybe change your diet.
But from Acupuncture to Zero Balancing
There's little difference and little gain,
So when you're done with them, or bored, or skint,
You could take this paper, moisten it,
Apply it as a poultice to the broken skin. Then wait
While meaning leaches through,
Performs its devious healing, remakes you.

Healing Spaces

Marguerite Bouvard

I have come to Provincetown, a tongue of land at the tip of Cape Cod, during a raw and chilly March. I will spend a week in the lower half of a house right on the water. The apartment is very dark, but there is a row of windows and a small jetty over the water where I am able to watch its moods, its changing textures and colors throughout days that are as seamless as the ocean. I watch the surge of high tide and wind-torn waves, listen to the rustle and slap of wavelets as the tide comes swishing in, and gaze at the pilings wavering in the sun-struck water.

Most days, I drive to Herring Cove where a strip of land serves as a parking lot directly in front of the beach. With the car facing the water, I turn off the motor and lean into the fierce expanse before me, the gull shadows racing over me. The ocean shuffles and reshuffles its deck in the splendor of its solitude and self-sufficiency. Nights, the ocean becomes black glass as sky and water dissolve into each other and the lighthouse flashes its beams through the windows.

I have come here to recover from a particularly bad bout of Interstitial Cystitis, an inflammation and deterioration of the bladder lining, and from weeks of acute pain and sleeplessness. Like a Zen hermit, I open the door of my house to the demons of weakness and despair, and allow the tears of frustration and exhaustion to well up like honored guests. I remember the words of my beloved colleague Ana when I was still able to work as a college professor and like a drunken Don Quixote flailed at all the injustices I perceived around me. "Oaks break, willows endure," she told me in her calm, gentle voice. Now her words return to me with new meaning: like the willow, I allow myself to bow beneath the wind, let my spirit graze earth, realizing that I also hold the sky. I allow time for the demons to walk about freely in the house, live my emotional pain so I can be strong again. I study the ocean as if it were a mirror revealing the person I have become, hemmed in by so many limitations and struggling to make a life for myself with an illness that is as unpredictable as it is debilitating.

In allowing my vulnerabilities to speak, I am also regenerating my spirit, giving myself the time to just be and trust that renewal will follow this letting go. An important part of healing is facing the tremendous anguish one endures during and after these bouts of acute symptoms. I often feel an overwhelming sense of powerlessness and sadness: these are not fleeting emotions, but feelings I need to traverse in solitude and over a stretch of time. These journeys bring me back to calmness and strength, for only in acknowledging and experiencing our own weakness can we become strong again. Perhaps because of a very deep-seated fear of both death and illness, there seems to be no room in our society for acknowledging such periods, which occur either after one has experienced a loss, or after a difficult time with an illness. They are invisible, but very rich moments when all our forces are marshaled and, although suffering, we are intensely focused and alive.

It has taken me many years to accept the person I have become since I came down with my illness in 1987. It began with nocturia and with my staggering through my days as a college professor in a drugged manner from lack of sleep. Since I had always been so healthy, I thought my problems were only passing and that I would return to my "normal state" in a matter of time. The fall after I was diagnosed, I hung on to my job in a state of complete denial. As the semester drew to a close, I knew I had to make some kind of adjustment and asked the president of the college if I could drop one course while retaining my committee and my advising. Even that didn't help, and the president then suggested that the sabbatical I was slated for might help relieve my symptoms. I never returned to that life. During the sabbatical, I traveled to Argentina briefly to work on a book about the Mothers of the Plaza de Mayo and that is when the bouts of spasms and intense pain began.

I left the planet of so-called normal people, who take for granted the ability to go through the days without overwhelming fatigue, and entered a new world. From a life as a professor, writer, activist, and parent, I moved into a world in which completing even a small task seemed overwhelming. I equate it to the period of disorganization that follows the numbness in the journey through grief. Ironically, I had written a book about loss, which appeared just before my illness struck. It never occurred to me that the loss of one's health is similar to the loss of a loved one.

During my sabbatical year, I had a fellowship at the Wellesley Center for Research on Women where I attended weekly seminars in a fog of exhaustion, listening to the conversations swirling around me as if behind a glass wall. My days which had once included exciting hours in the classroom, conducting research in the library, and attending professional events seemed to have shrunk. I stayed at home, struggling to sit at my desk while working on the book about the Mothers and taking long naps in the afternoon.

I can now tell people who inquire about me, it's different than it once was, but it's a life. Although I have created an intense and satisfying way of being, I am still subject to a roller coaster of physical and emotional jolts. While I have periods of feeling as well as possible under the circumstances, I also tunnel through weeks of utter darkness: I am like Lazarus, rising repeatedly within myself. After such periods, I turn to nature, to its calming pace, losing myself in a world that transcends our small egos and my own frailty. In society, my limitations often seem to relegate me to the margins; here I become part of the ocean's vast expanses.

As so many of the difficulties that are an inextricable part of life's passages, illness is an invitation to explore the inner spaces, the depths of ourselves and our possibilities. In so doing I invent new ways of living with my situation and have discovered meaning. This is an ongoing process and for me occurs both during my daily meditation and the long periods of time I spend alone. Battling my condition is very demanding of the soul. Sometimes I feel like an overburdened ox plodding from one end of the field to another, for suffering is often tedious and very much like a job without hours. Other times, it brings me closer to illuminations, for meditation gives me a sense of perspective and, above all, of spaciousness. When I meditate, my boundaries and limitations melt away. Sometimes powerful images come to me.

I remember the last trip I took to Argentina to work on the book about the Mothers of the Plaza de Mayo. I worried whether I could handle the long journey and the stress and dangers of the work, for the Mothers and their supporters are continually harassed by the security forces. I was meditating one afternoon, shortly before going to Argentina, when I had a vision of myself standing in a crowded subway holding onto a strap. Looking up, I noticed that the supporting bar was made of solid light. That image made little sense to me until I was in the throes of working with the Mothers and experienced a remission. For two weeks I was pain free and able to spend my days without napping, although I went to bed exhausted at eight o'clock every night.

During my daily meditations, I have developed the habit of reviewing the day, of counting the blessings I have experienced—such as a phone call from a friend or a period of two hours of writing, which is a rare and great gift. I have learned how precious life is and to cherish the instances of joy each day brings. Before my illness, I tended to notice what was missing rather than what was there and only waiting for me to acknowledge it. Now, I have come to see the presence of the Creator shining in what may seem like the most ordinary events of daily life.

Spending time in the wondrous presence of the ocean is like a long meditation. I leave behind the world where one is supposed to be "doing" and where one is measured by one's productivity. Here in Provincetown, I try to suspend judgment on myself because I am unable to work. I take the day as if I were a child again and let time flow around me like the surge of waves.

Mornings, I write in my journal, noting both the beauty around me and recording the storms within. It is an important space, for these pages are uncensored and I can pour myself out freely. As someone who is chronically ill, I constantly mask my feelings in order not to burden family and friends. I have kept a journal since the early days of my illness and have found that it has many uses—as a room where my true self can unfold, a place to record my discoveries, to vent my frustration, and ultimately as a way of reviewing the great distances I have traveled. Outside my window the endless reweaving of the surf seems to mirror the pages of my diary. It is where I come to know myself and gain a deeper understanding of life.

I also take long walks through the narrow streets and I walk with my whole being, observing the routines of the town—the high-school youngsters tumbling out of school, the elderly sitting on benches and chatting, the young mothers with strollers. Breathing in the tangy sea air, I forget the lists of things to do we all carry in our heads. There is nothing but the wind, the ocean, and the privacy of a small town resort out of season, the present as infinite as the ocean. Buddhists would refer to such complete attention to the moment as *mindfulness.* I have learned to savor life slowly, not to rush through the day so intent upon accomplishment that I miss the many facets of what may seem at first sight like insignificant times. It is a way of mining the life around me.

As the week draws to a close, I have regained my sense of serenity. Watching the ocean, the walls vanish as I am caught up in its moods and shifting hues. I breathe in its vastness and its intimacy, reminding myself that I have relinquished neither despite my daily battles. If at times it seems as if I am being forced by my illness into an ever-smaller space, a prison within a prison, I can always look at the ocean and see myself journeying within the boundless reaches of our common humanity and the inexhaustible spaces of the heart.

My Visualization

Varda Nowack Goldstein

Close your eyes, relax . . . Imagine you are at the top of a staircase. I will count backwards from 10 as you descend the stairs. 10-9-8 . . .

The staircase is always the same. This is my favorite place on earth. I have entered it through a carved oak door. Above the door it reads OZ. As I come through the doorway I see a small, white stone Buddha seated on a smooth, carved bench. A polished stone rests in the Buddha's lap. Truth, it reads. Some days it reads Faith, and other days it reads Acceptance.

I descend the winding, trellised staircase, turning as I move down. On my right the stone path weaves towards a wooden picket gate. I know that behind that gate a narrow stone bridge spans a tangled canyon of wild flowers and ancient trees. I imagine the deep grooved canyon worn by ages of rainwater rushing toward the Pacific. The other end of the bridge is guarded by another low gate. And beyond that a ramp and more stairs twist and turn toward the two-story guesthouse perched at the canyon's edge.

As I move down the staircase I can look to my left and see an English garden, vibrant in a spring burst of yellows, pinks, blues, and violet laid against a riot of green. A rope swing hangs from a mammoth redwood tree, swinging in the breeze toward a delicate wood table with two small benches. A copper teapot sits in the middle of the table waiting for the inevitable warm spell. The main house is beyond—an A-frame of wood and glass.

On my good days I walk straight ahead from the stairs, meandering through rows of wild flowers and kitchen spices. The crushed-rock path leads me to another stone bench on which another solemn Buddha sits and contemplates the small altar of candles before a statue of Jesus. I stop and light a votive candle, more as a thank you for the beauty of this place than as a prelude for prayer.

The sun is high in the sky. From the small altar I can see the distant Pacific undulating in varied stripes of blue, sky and ocean blended in a lightening stripe.

Jesus, the Buddha, and I are small against the panorama of endless sky and never-ending sea. There is no sound. The hawks are napping, drowsy in the intensity of light. Insects burrow deep in the brush, aware of summer just beyond their wings. Occasionally the wind blows across the canyon. It is cold and damp, filled with salt and brine. I embrace the sun and imagine each ray seeping through my body, confirming health.

On my bad days, I descend from the entrance and walk quickly past my stone friends to descend another stairway of stone rubbed smooth by rain, wind, and winter. Weeds peek up through the ragged log frame surrounding each step. I fight to retain my balance, for here there are no railings.

I am always surprised that at the bottom of these steep steps there is a meadow of ordered grass and neatly trimmed bushes. The sauna is to my right, the potter's shed and swimming pool to my left.

From the meadow fence, I see below me the canyon running in dense forest to the ribbon of pale ocean. The fog is thick in places, allowing me only an occasional glimpse of water. I close my eyes and slowly raise my arms. In the air I can hear mermaids singing their mournful siren song to long-lost Spanish galleons beached and sunk along the ragged Monterey coast.

"Allah Akbar, God is Great," the Arabic words spring from within me. "Adonai Malak, God is King," an ancient Hebrew prayer continues.

I am Eve, banished from Eden, now returned to pray for my life. "Forgive me Father, for I have sinned," I say.

The wind winds around me and whispers, "I who know your heart have long since forgiven."

My arms toward heaven, I prepare to ask for my life, but from deep within my soul I surrender and simply pray, "Into Thy hands I commend my soul. Thy will be done."

I am going to count back from 10. When you hear 3 you will slowly awake, rested and peaceful and ready to go on with your day.

The Pilgrimage

Madeleine Parish

The first time I went to France, in 1991, I packed a duffel bag full of black and gray Joan Vass knits, my Nikon, my journal. I took my limited but well-rehearsed French vocabulary and my late-blooming wanderlust. I was thirty-nine. I went by limo, alone, to Kennedy Airport, ate croissants and Brie en route, stayed in the eighteenth arondissement at a studio apartment. I wanted to come back saying I had discovered something new about myself when I saw the Monet collection at the D'Orsay, experienced higher truth while meditating on the rose windows at Chartres, and that I had been inspired to creative heights at Stendahl's grave. When I returned from my ten-day tour, I brought back journal entries and photos, a pink and yellow silk Hermes scarf, Chanel Numero Cinque for my mother, coffee table books from the Louvre, and my first symptoms of Chronic Fatigue Syndrome.

Five years later, on my next trip to France, I am taking a charter flight full of people who, like me, are sick and want to get well. Some have cancer. Some can't see. Some can't walk. Some talk in single syllables most of us can't understand, while their bodies jerk and twist in steely wheelchairs. Again, I pack my duffel with well-coordinated knits, but this time I take my illness, my hope, my despair, my fear. I leave behind my camera and journal. I have no room for observation on this trip. I want only one thing: to be cured at Lourdes, where the mother of Christ appeared over a hundred years ago in a gray stone grotto to a fourteen-year-old farm girl named Bernadette. And where millions go each year to bathe in the waters that sprang up on the spot were Mary appeared and to pray for miraculous healing in their own imperfect lives.

* * *

Our pilgrimage starts from Kennedy Airport on May 1, 1996, but the journey that led me to Lourdes began months earlier. By April 1995, when my illness left me so weak and disoriented I could no longer work, I began going to Mass on the mornings I could get out of bed.

On the first sunny Saturday in March 1996, I was tempted to pray while I turned over dirt and picked up limp twigs and matted brown leaves in my garden. It had been a long, hard winter, with record-breaking snowfall for much of the Northeast and near spirit-breaking pain and frustration for me. I wanted to touch the earth, plug into the current that was waking my hostas and astilbe and stargazer lilies from their winter sleep. If I could connect with the force that was resurrecting my garden, I thought, maybe I could come to life again, too.

I couldn't afford to take chances—maybe this would be the day I would be cured—so I went to church. At the end of the half hour, when I spent more time thinking where I might transplant pachysandra than about whether Christ died to redeem sin, a woman approached me as I turned to leave my regular pew.

Her name was Hope, she said. She had heard I was ill and wanted to know how I was feeling.

"Up and down," I told her, and with her next breath she said she was organizing a pilgrimage to Lourdes.

"Do you want to go?" she asked.

Maybe it doesn't show, I thought in the small space between her question and my answer—the fact that I come here every day, not because I am faithful, but because I am filled with fear. That I take my seat next to women who follow the Mass with well worn leather-bound missals, who move their lips in silent steady prayer, because I will try anything, hocus pocus or systematically documented scientific fact, anything that might help me get well.

"I appreciate the opportunity," I said, "But I can't afford it." I looked away, embarrassed.

"We'll pay," she said.

I wrestled with my thoughts. Lourdes was somewhere shrinking Italian grandmothers with arthritis went, wasn't it? Still, I had tried daily injections of experimental drugs, gluten-free diets, homeopathy.

"Yes," I said. I would go to Lourdes because I wanted to get well more than I wanted to not believe, more than I was concerned about looking needy or foolish.

* * *

Off and on, until I board the 747 headed for France, I'm skeptical. I want proof. So I go to Borders bookstore to read up on Lourdes. "Every year," I read in one well-regarded travel guide, "more than five million pilgrims head to Lourdes searching for miraculous cures. Whether it's worth the trip is another matter." The surrounding area, the book says, is listless, and the town itself, packed with more hotel rooms than any French city except Paris, is littered with shops hawking rosaries with beads the size of ping pong balls, and translucent lawn ornaments in likenesses of Mary and Christ.

I leave Borders with questions swarming like hornets 'round my head. Am I out of my mind? Chasing windmills? Will my doctors (both Jewish) think me a fool? (No, as a matter of fact, they both say I must go, I must do whatever might help me get well.)

At the library, I read Gothic tales of sixty-four cures at Lourdes, documented over recent decades by both medical authorities and the Church. A British soldier, paralyzed by wounds incurred at Gallipoli, left Lourdes in 1923 pushing the wheelchair he had arrived in. Two decades later, a French woman with a baseball-sized uterine tumor arrived in Lourdes on a stretcher and walked away, days later, cancer-free. If they went to Lourdes broken, and if they returned whole, could the same thing happen to me?

Faith comes and goes. At Mass pesky questions skinny through its cracks like mice scratching in a wall. When I hold the Eucharistic wafer in my palm, I think this can't possibly be the body of Christ. Or can it? And how can I pray to the Blessed Mother, who, in her purity and gentleness, has always seemed so elusive and distant? Now with Mary Magdalene I could at least find common ground. I know how she felt when she visited the tomb after Christ was taken there, how she wouldn't go away until she found out where He went. But the other Mary? The real Mary? What would we talk about besides the weather, the price of fish?

I review my scorecard as a sometime Catholic and assess the odds, given my spotty commitment over the years, on whether I can find a place in the Church. Or, for that matter, whether I can take a seat on the plane next to my fellow pilgrims.

* * *

On May 1, my friend Al drives me to the airport. We pray in the car on the way—for him, for me, for his brother-in-law with cancer, for other friends. After we park the car and go into the terminal, he hands my bag to a man named Jack, someone I have never met or spoken to. I want to run back to Al's car with him. But Jack takes my arm before I can turn away and introduces me to his wife Carol and to other pilgrims: Debbie, a twelve-yearold paraplegic who wheels around in a motorized chair; Susan, a forty-three-year-old mother with two children and breast cancer; Tim, an eight-year-old with cerebral palsy and a mother whose name might have been Patience.

Jack introduces me to members of the organization that sponsored the trip—wealthy Catholics with a mission to help the sick and the poor. I recognize some of them or their names, at least, from what I have read about them and their accomplishments in *The Wall Street Journal* or *The Washington Post.* Does it show, I wonder, the anger, the embarrassment I feel that I am on the needy side of this equation? I hope not.

Jack and Carol become my helpers for the week. They get me on the plane in New York, and off again when we descend the next morning, through a dramatic purple sky into the farmland at the foot of the Pyrenees in the southwest corner of France.

The tour books are right, I think, when we drive into town. Hotels the equivalents of Days Inns and Howard Johnson Motor Lodges are wedged into every available land parcel, and, except for the mauvish haze over the mountains, and the red and blue and green fluorescent hotel signs, the town is gray: from the cloud cover so thick it seems painted, to the convents' and hospitals' stone facades, to the cobblestone streets underfoot. "Whether it's worth the trip is another matter." The words I had read in the tour book surface and doubt knocks hope out of position and regains solid position. How can healing take place, how can health be affirmed against this lifeless gray scrim? I try to look like I am anxious to get on with the healing, but inside my heart sinks. I check into my little room with the narrow bed. I open the French doors that look out over the gray river flowing across the street, but I see no sign of possibility. I try to nap, but sleep escapes me and I want to go home.

My fellow pilgrims and I number about two hundred. That afternoon we arrive in Lourdes, and each of the next six days we line up in front of our hotel and process to the Grotto. Carol and Jack wheel me in a cart called a *voiture.* It takes all my strength to allow this attention. I am used to going it alone.

We are joined by thousands of other pilgrims from all over the world, walking toward the Grotto, walking, we hope, toward health. Traffic stops whenever a group of malades (as we infirm pilgrims are called) is escorted through town. We are afforded other courtesies as well: the best seats at Masses, the opportunity to receive the Eucharist before the others. We are, we are told, honored guests, entitled because of our frailties to places of high regard. I don't want to insult my hosts, but the price of admission for this honor has been too great. I would gladly trade my front row seat for the ability to stand up, smile graciously, and walk away, whole and self-reliant once again.

* * *

The Grotto is dull and gray, ordinary, and disappointing—a mass of stone only a couple stories high, with a dwarfish statue of the Blessed Mother wedged in a crevice. Candles are placed at her feet and lighted by pilgrims parading by. Crutches and braces are left there, too, discarded by people who no longer need them because Mary has interceded in their lives. Signs, I want to believe, that this place might offer hope after all.

We pilgrims parade together wherever we go: to Mass for twenty thousand, said in six languages, in an underground cathedral the size of Shea Stadium; to healing services held around the banks of the river that flows next to the imposing Basilica near the Grotto. Clergy sweep past in robes that swirl in the wind around their feet. Priests in black defer to bishops in fuchsia, bishops to cardinals in red. Among us are Italian women wearing fine silks and excessive gold; big Polish men with swollen stomachs and noses, like the men I grew up around; Irish men with no limbs pushed by red-headed teenagers with curls flaming away from their freckled faces. It is in this stream of life, of many moving together, that I feel the first possibility, the first offer, of health.

Each evening thousands of us march around the Basilica courtyard carrying lighted candles, forming one long river of hope and light. We sing together, pray together, as the sun lowers orange and round behind the buttresses that root the church in the soil. Some of us sing in English, some in French, some in Polish. Some pray with moving lips but no sounds come from them. We don't need to understand or even hear each other's words, though, to understand each other's purpose.

An Italian woman swoons, then curls like a cat on the ground. We call for help; she must be ill, we think. No, her husband assures us. The spirit sometimes does this to her. What spirit, I wonder. Could a spirit that knocks a woman's legs out from under her be trusted? I'm not sure. But when I look behind me and see us marching together and when I hear us singing together, polite and kind, though different, I believe that if heaven waits for us, it must look and feel and sound like this.

* * *

I put off going to the baths until the day before we are to leave Lourdes, mostly because I'm afraid the disappointment might be unbearable if I don't walk out of the water healthy and whole. I also want time to prepare properly, to do everything I can to make healing possible. That means praying, resting, going to confession. Since I have not received the sacrament of reconciliation for many years, I want to find a priest, the right priest, who will judge me least and comfort me most.

In the dining room, over lunch, I evaluate the possibilities. I eliminate the clergy who seem most comfortable in the Church hierarchy: the Richard Chamberlain look-alike currently on loan to Rome from the Bishop's office, or the red-faced Irishman who leads us in Broadway show tunes after dinner each night. I skip over any of them under age forty, anyone who wears his black cassock too well, anyone too pious, too jovial, too guarded, too stern.

I see a man of sixty or so sitting two tables away. He wears a black suit and clerical collar, and he's pushed himself from the table. His plate is not clean, but he's had enough. His hands are folded atop his full stomach.

A kindly, closed-mouth smile warms his shiny, reddish face while he listens to others at his table. He speaks little, he nods, he smiles.

Father Banks is from Los Angeles, Carol tells me when I ask about him, and on Sunday afternoons he heads into dark neighborhoods and hands out dollars to men and women who live in boxes or on benches.

"He was stabbed once," she says, "by a man with a knife and no home. But he still goes back." I could trust a man with that smile, I think. Someone who has been hurt and can return to the place where he bled and try again.

I approach Father Banks as the dining room clears. "Will you hear my confession?" I ask. And when he extends his arm and his smile and motions toward a stuffed sofa in the lobby I wish instead for the dark safe distance of the tall mahogany confessional closets of my childhood—a dimly lit place where I can walk in, leave my anonymous sins in the darkness, and walk out. Instead I sit next to him on a sofa.

He smiles and nods, and I start slowly, carefully. "Bless me Father, for I have sinned." The words are distant, difficult at first for me to pull up after years of neglect, but when they come, they feel familiar and surprisingly safe. I continue in the fluorescent light of that public place, working my way past the smaller transgressions, to the worst of what I have to say: that I can find no love from or for the God that allows this sickness, this latest obstacle.

Father Banks listens. He is still. When I am through talking, I look at him and see that his eyes are closed. His breath is deep and slow. He is waiting, it seems, not for the words he might want to say, but the words he is intended to say. "I believe," he says finally, "that I am asked to tell you that you would not have been brought to this holy place, this healing place, if you were not loved, if you were not invited to grace and health and reconciliation."

What had I heard since I was a child in the Church, if not that Christ died for my sins? That my sins were forgiven through Him. And why is it that, until this moment, I have been willing to believe it might be true for others, but not for me? I want at first to ask, "Is it true for me, too?" But when I look into his eyes, they are rooted in such gentleness I am willing to believe. I can take the gift offered through this man. I say the closing prayers, and he raises his hand above me and makes the sign of the cross.

"I bless you in the name of the Father," he says as I look up at the hand, "and the Son." Is this the hand that was stabbed and healed, the wound that was healed in order that this man might better heal others? "And the Holy Spirit," he says. And in that moment, I am willing to believe for the first time that I can be forgiven, that I can heal.

* * *

Carol and I walk to the baths in the flat stone building just beyond the Grotto. I take my place next to other women each waiting her turn on a sagging wooden bench in a hallway with a cold cement floor. A woman calls me to go behind a curtain, blue, the color of the Blessed Mother. I take off my clothes with the other women with other illnesses, hurts, disappointments, and fears, and a French woman wraps me in a blue sheet. She takes me behind the next curtain and I stand in front of the stone bath, which is long, narrow, gray, and frightening because it is the size and shape of a crypt. A woman with kindness in her eyes leads me to the foot of the bath, and when I take the first step down, the water up to my ankles, my breath stops. The water is too cold. I turn toward the woman. I can go no further.

"Breathe," she says. "Breathe!" I take air into my throat, my chest, my stomach as best I can. "Walk to the end of the bath," the woman says. "Then touch the statue of the Blessed Mother and make your intention to her."

I walk, feeling as if I am no longer under my own power. Is it the cold? Is it the spirit that made the Italian woman swoon while we paraded around the Basilica? I don't know, but I walk through the water, up to my calves. "Hail Mary, full of grace." The women pray out loud with me. I walk to the end of the bath and I become confused. I want to get well. I want to get well, Mary. But I want not to be alone. Should I ask for a husband? Can I have him and my health, too? Do I need him more than I need my health? Is it too much to ask? It is only a short walk, ten or twelve steps, but my mind moves faster than my feet. I reach the end of the bath. I touch the image of Mary.

"My health," I say. "Please. Help me get well."

I turn and walk back, no longer cold. My body vibrates, like a hot light is shining inside me, pulsing. The women help me get out of the bath. After I dry myself and dress, I meet Carol and we walk back to the hotel in silence.

* * *

The next day, we board our plane and head back to New York. Some of us still cannot see. Some of us still thrash in wheelchairs and drool down our chins. My body still hurts and I am still groggy with fatigue. I am not cured. I am different though, relieved of the burden of disbelief, knowing for the first time that my sins are forgiven. I have been healed, through my body to my spirit, gifted with restorative grace, hope, and faith. I can move forward, expectant of continued love. And I am not alone.

A Grateful Cancer Survivor

Molly Ivins

In one week and two days, I will be finished with nine months of treatment for cancer. First they poison you; then they mutilate you; then they burn you. I've had more fun. And when it's almost over, you're so glad that you're grateful to absolutely everyone. And I am.

We've all done our best here; whether this thing comes back is out of all of our hands. My wise friend Marlyn Schwartz said that those of us who survive owe a debt—to Carole Kneeland, Mary Sherrill, Jocelyn Gray and all the others who didn't make it. They would have given anything they owned, any part of their bodies, for the gift of life. We who survive have it, and we owe it to them to cherish it—joyfully.

The trouble is, I'm not a better person. I was in great hopes that confronting my own mortality would make me deeper, more thoughtful. Many lovely people sent books on how to find a deeper spiritual meaning in life. My response was, "Oh, hell, I can't go on a spiritual journey—I'm constipated."

Being sick actually narrows your world, I'm afraid—makes you focus more on yourself. Maybe when it's over and you don't feel like crud all the time, then your spirit soars. The chief reason to keep working is because it takes your mind off yourself.

The main thing they tell you, over and over, is that

this is different for everyone. Everyone reacts differently to chemotherapy, to surgery, to radiation.

I vomited in the office, couldn't sleep forever, lost 50 pounds. I don't recommend the diet. I was like, "Help, I'm flunking cancer."

Of course, I laughed a lot—who could not laugh? There's even a cancer-humor Web site called "Tarry, Black Stools." I got my first hair a few weeks ago. It came in right next to my mouth—that little moustache I've always hated. That God—what a sense of humor.

Before surgery, my friend Mercedes Pena decided that I needed to get in touch with my emotions. I'd just as soon not hear from my emotions; I suspect that they're largely unpleasant. A long-distance call once or twice a year is enough for me.

But Mercy insisted. Sure enough, I was not happy about having a radical mastectomy. I said, "Mercy, how in the world do you Latinas do this every day, all the time in touch with the emotions?"

She said seriously, "That's why we take siestas."

Cancer is good for the priorities. Traffic, for one thing, is not worth getting upset about. As my pal Spike Gillespie says, you look at those fools honking, getting steamed, cutting in front of you and you just think, "Hey, it's not a malignant tumor, you know?"

You can't get through this without a lot of help from your friends. I had a party for all my helpers after I got through with chemo. It's hard for me to talk about things that I care deeply about without at least trying to be funny, but I told them how much they mean to me. The value of that friendship is so much greater than any of the suffering caused by cancer that it's not even remotely close.

Despite my request, untold numbers of people wrote wonderful cards, notes, letters. My friends sent funny stuff by e-mail. I'd save it up, and about once a month when I couldn't sleep at 3 a.m., I'd be sitting in front of the computer, laughing and laughing. And I'm most grateful of all to the women who went out and got mammograms.

And that brings us to another great benefit of the Big C. It's the world's greatest excuse. I've gotten out of more stuff I didn't want to do—even more than the stuff I missed that I did want to do.

Cancer is not easy, it is not pleasant, and given a choice, I would just as soon have skipped it. But I now know what all survivors know, and I am grateful. So grateful.

I Dreamt of an Arm

Felicia Ferlin

Most nights, sleep is a vast, precious world of denial. My dreams are rich and unburdened, subject only to the peculiar limits of the subconscious: I spy behind enemy lines in occupied France; night-surf the Pacific guarded by fireflies; I even sit painlessly for hours, bantering with friends over too much wine and too many courses. I am whole, and the world of sleep is infinite in its realm of possibility.

Last night, however, I dreamt of the first time—the worst time. I dreamt of loss, of reaching into a box in a dark, hollow room. I dreamt of sliding fingers and opposing thumb around the cool, smooth binding of a book whose title I cannot remember. What I do remember is an arm suddenly become foreign, a grasp so separated that it became inanimate. Dead, the arm refused to obey. The book slipped back to wedge itself among the other books where, like me, it felt it belonged nestled safely among the memories of the life I'd loved so very much. At that moment, the life I thought I could bring to the West Coast fell back to bury itself in one of the many unpacked boxes still moldering in my garage.

Throughout the day, I wear my dreams. If the dreams are good, I am decorated with courage and potential; if bad, I am smeared by pain and weakness. Today's markings do not bode well, but I resolve to wear them all day.

This is important as I move forward—as I prepare for the next version of my life.

Change is cumbersome. Change tries even the most whole among us. My subconscious forces me to pry my grief loose, but my loss of dexterity sends it flying. Regardless, I must honor the dark, hollow room. I must walk across its cold wooden floor to that box. I must find a way to reach in and pull the grief close to my chest. To move forward, I must go back to the beginning—back to what was then, the end.

Seven years have passed since I betrayed my arms. Seven years since they, in turn, betrayed me. I've had a long time to learn about myself and this condition. During this time, I've grown much stronger. Grief, however, is enough of a burden for one day. If I've learned anything from any of this, I've learned to respect my limits.

Today I will wear my grief, but looking forward takes hope—and the weight of that will have to wait for a different day.

Pas de Deux with Mister D

Adan Williams

It was January 1986 when I learned that I had contracted HIV, the retrovirus that leads to AIDS. I had turned twenty five just a few weeks earlier, in late November of the previous year. The news hit me like a visceral thud, as if the rug of my relatively comfortable life had been pulled out from under me, both rudely and abruptly. Unlike the men dying of AIDS in the news, I had not had thousands, hundreds, or even half a dozen sex partners, and my drug use, far from any habitual or addictive chemical dependency, was limited to an occasional toke of marijuana with high school and college friends over the years. I didn't even smoke cigarettes; and if there was any substance to which I was addicted at the time, it was probably carrot juice.

The counselor at the Los Angeles Gay and Lesbian Center's new HIV testing unit broke the news in sterile stride, her matter-of-fact tone chilling my soul. "Your test came back positive. It says here, 'light exposure.' I've never seen that before. You may want to come back and be tested again just to be certain." I was stunned—shocked. A single tear rolled down my cheek. The urge to protest, to insist there must be some mistake, was stifled by the flood of countless confused feelings that rushed up and overtook the purely self-assertive defiance of the initial impulse. I had gone into the clinic two weeks before to put what I felt were irrational fears behind me. So many nights I had lain awake in bed groping under my arms, around my groin, along my throat, wondering if my glands were swollen. Even though my doctor assured me my glands were normal, I needed to be certain that I was free and clear of this strange new virus.

I remember clearly the surreal haze I walked in that day, like a somnambulist, as I made my way back to my car. Parked at the corner of De Longpre and Highland, I sat in the driver's seat and stared blankly into the rear view mirror. Evening rush hour traffic filed by as usual in a smog-enshrouded stream of honking horns and blinking lights: nothing seemed to have changed in the life of Hollywood, but I reeled in the realization that nothing in my own life would be the same again. I felt at once betrayed and lost, humbled and scared. I felt ashamed. Mostly I felt that, without even knowing it, I had somehow thrown away the sweet life I had been given, had wasted the investments of love and hope my parents and grandparents, even my aunts, uncles, and sisters and cousins had made in me. Amazingly, I was already missing my family, already sensing the grief they would all experience watching my slow demise as disease after opportunistic disease ravaged my young body. In the days to come I would hear my doctor say, "In two years you can expect to be very, very sick. And I'm afraid you'll never see your thirtieth birthday." And yet, sitting there in my car, I had no sense of being in my body at all. My consciousness had radically shifted, and what I had once understood to be a secure reality no longer had any ground to stand on. My mind and my heart were as much adrift in a sea of uncertainty as they were uncommonly estranged from one another.

The sudden impulse to stage a protest arose again, but this time with greater clarity and passion. It felt like the old Black Power days of the 60s and 70s, only with this difference: It was not a white man but a white coat that I would not let dictate my fate to me. I simply was not ready to die. It was crystal clear to me, like looking into a magic mirror and seeing the truth for the first time, that at twenty five my life had just begun, that I had not even begun to live yet, and that I wanted very much to live the life that, as recently as two hours before, I imagined lay ahead of me. Insisting that the common belief about AIDS need not be true for me—the belief that AIDS spelled a certain death—I prayed to God that I be shown a way to thrive in the face of all the news and talk around me, despite that media-stream of negativity meant only to convince me and every one else that I was doomed to die in a gruesome way.

Lost in my prayer, an inner light broke through my fear. Silence pregnant with a deeper reality shined forth, and the still voice of that silence spoke to me, saying, "Your life doesn't end here, son. Here is where your life's true work begins."

Something inside me quickened as I turned the car's ignition. "Curiosity killed the cat," I said with defiant confidence. "But the cat has nine lives." This became my first mantra, and I repeated it for years, albeit in the form of a reconciliatory prayer. "Om namah shivaya" is my mantra today, sacred syllables given to me by my spiritual teacher, meaning: "I honor the Lord who dwells within me." This is the mantra I credit today with saving my life and sustaining my being.

Upon my diagnosis, I realized it was time to change my

tune. I had studied yoga and Vedanta, two ancient philosophies of India, and I also remembered how once, after reading the Bhagavad-Gita, I tried repeating the sacred mantra "Hare Krishna Hare Ram," and the whole room lit up perceptibly around me. If a mantra could change my external environment in such a profound way, I saw even greater implications for my internal environment as well. I remembered something I learned about karma as well—the law of action and reaction: heartfelt positive effort consistently and assiduously applied in the present can lessen and even nullify the results of negative karma from past actions. "Love is stronger than death," I'd read in Solomon's ancient song, and I believed him.

I developed a new understanding: "The more I love and invest in life, the more life will love and invest in me." I wanted to fill my life with living from the heart. Instead of expecting more and more from what I once believed life owed me, I decided to give up on my attachment to lifelong self-centered dreams of wealth and fame. I surrendered my fledgling career in motion picture production to became a schoolteacher, hoping to share with others some of the bounty that my heart had already received. (I have now lived long enough to see at least one of my junior high students go on to become a high school teacher himself.) In time I also began to support local reforestation projects, donating my sweat, my muscle, and my dollars to developing and sustaining a healthier Los Angeles. (Now when I drive along a once bare concrete and asphalt covered stretch of Robertson Boulevard, I see the dozens of beautiful trees I helped plant shading the storefronts and passersby.) All this is to say that I have now lived long enough to see some kind of positive legacy resulting from my own desire to live a healthy life and survive a cold death sentence I was not prepared to take.

I also affirmed my life by seeing the world. If I had to die before thirty, I wanted to see Spain and Italy again. I also wanted to visit India, Japan, and the French Antilles before I went. The last trip I took abroad, however, significantly changed my perspective on death and dying, and on life and living.

In 1992 I had an extraordinary dream wherein I was shown I would find a brick of gold on a beautiful tropical island. At one end of the island there rose a majestic green volcano, and at the foot of the volcano a vast field of sun-ripening, redolent pineapples spread out as far as the eye could see. In the dream, once I had this gold in hand, I had the conviction that it was not for me alone, but more importantly it was mine to share with all who needed it. As hauntingly beautiful and promising as it was, this was truly an impenetrably mysterious dream. Then, three years later in the summer of 1995, by a series of curiously arising circumstances, I landed on the island of Martinique where something rather remarkable happened.

Already my life story had outlived by five years the deadline it was given, but even so I was still living with the nagging idea that an early death was dancing on my heels. My parents had suggested I go to the Caribbean island of Saint Martin and spend a week or two. They had in mind buying a vacation home there and thought perhaps I'd like to live on the island year round. The relatively stress-free environment, they wagered, would be good for my health. To discern whether this was a good idea, I agreed to take a trip.

Indeed, it had been nine years since my original diagnosis, and even though subsequent testing had shown that my "light exposure" was still considered enough to land me six feet under, I hadn't developed any AIDS-related opportunistic infections. Over the years my doctors said to me again and again, "Whatever it is you're doing, just keep doing it." Island life sounded like the next best thing to a true panacea for what ailed me.

When I arrived in Saint Martin I knew right away that I could never live there. The whole island catered to a brand of hedonism I found unsettling. Casinos, boutiques, and beach-concealing hotels abounded, and this was far from any place I thought I'd like to call home. Recognizing that my precious vacation dollars were being ill-spent in that place, I hastened to a bookstore to investigate other islands I could visit with my remaining money. Leafing through a big book full of color photos, I turned a page and my wide eyes landed on a vast field of pineapples above which rose a majestic green volcano! My consciousness exploded, seemed to expand beyond the bounds of my skin and fill the entire store. I lost my breath, but when I caught it again I looked at the photo more closely. It was without doubt the island from my dream! At the top of the page the heading read, Martinique. The next day I was on a plane heading to that extraordinary haven.

After landing, the cabbie from the airport asked me why I, an American, had chosen to come to Martinique, not the most popular vacation destination for Americans. I explained to him that I had had a dream of pineapples under a green volcano, and when I saw the photograph in the bookstore the day before, I knew that there was something waiting for me on his island.

"Well, if you want to see pineapples, monsieur," he said, "take a van up Mount Pelee. From there you will see all the pineapple fields you want!"

The next day I caught a van up the slope of the great volcano, Mount Pelee. As suggested by my cabbie, I stopped off in a town called Morne Rouge. Entering the street I was halted in my tracks by an unsurpassable beauty unlike any I had seen in any other part of the world. Mist-enshrouded peaks bearing tall stands of bamboo littered every hillside, and bright red flowers cascaded all around them. The main road was peopled with loving mothers and children speaking sweetly to one another. The people of Martinique had a kind of breezy, smooth bearing, a stress-free way of being in their bodies that betrayed a deep comfort with themselves and their surroundings, something all but missing, I felt, in African Americans—including myself. I was enveloped by what must have been the most beautiful scene I'd ever laid eyes on, and tears soon welled up in my eyes.

Something about this scene touched deep inside my heart. It caressed with a healing hand all the places where American racism had wounded me, the places I had become numb to, and which, having taken them so long for granted, I no longer even realized existed. The people here it seemed were supremely free of the stress of racism. They were not angry. There was no strife or any sign of violence on the street. In its place there was great joy. Joy in the eyes of the passing mothers. Joy in the laughter of their children by their sides. Joy in the voices of the workmen. And overall simplicity.

I sat down under a tree and cried quiet, bittersweet tears. I was happy to see black people like this, and at the same time I felt a strange, bitter resentment. I resented having had to live always questioning my humanity, my equality, going out of my way to make others feel comfortable around me. How many times had white women clutched their purses when I entered an elevator or approached them on the street? How many times had I tried to walk in a non-threatening way to disarm their fears? What did that dance ultimately do to me, editing my every public move? Though I might be thinking of how pretty the birds sounded singing in the trees above my head, invariably someone would look at me and remind me that I was already guilty of crimes they'd only imagined, a natural born hardened criminal. Until now I had never realized just how much this sad dance had hurt me over the thirty four years of my life.

A ginger-colored man emerged from a neighboring building and asked me what was wrong. Tall, well-built and handsome, I looked at him in awe. "I am from the United States," I explained. "I've never experienced a place as beautiful as this. The happy people . . ."

He invited me back to his office and asked why I had chosen to come to Morne Rouge of all places. I said I was looking for a field of pineapples that I had seen in a dream three years before. Just then a voice rang out from behind me. "Bonjour, Papa!" I turned and saw the most radiant face I think I had ever seen on a child. And what's more, the boy looked like me, a "me" undefiled by the poison of homophobic taunts and the smallness that results from fighting to remain civil in the face of incivility, of hoping to be seen as an equal, of struggling to neatly uproot and dispose of far too many angry race-based sentiments.

"Adan," said Marcel, "I'd like for you to meet my son, Gregory. Gregory, say hello to Adan." The boy smiled a sweet smile my way. His father asked him to take me to the only pineapple field around Morne Rouge. Gregory protested at first but at last complied, and the next thing I knew we were climbing fences, dodging a bull, uprooting herbs for tea, throwing rocks in the quarry, and yanking down grapefruits from fruit-laden trees. When finally we reached the pineapple field just outside of town, I realized it was not pineapples I had come to find. I saw that my gold was this child with the most beautiful golden eyes, my own unwounded inner self standing before me, healthy, happy and free.

When finally Gregory and I returned to his father, Marcel invited me to go back to my hotel and pack my things. "You will return to Morne Rouge and stay with us tomorrow, and for as long as you'd like." I agreed.

That night under the full moonlight, I went swimming in a secluded cove. I had taken a walk long and far away from my hotel, and I hadn't brought a swimsuit with me. So when I chanced upon the hidden cove, I stripped down to my bare skin and dove right in. The moon's light illumined the cove and the two hillsides that spilled down into it. The water was so clear, and the moonlight so bright, that I was able to stand waist deep in the cove and still see the hairs on my toes. It was truly an amazing experience.

Suddenly overcome with tremendous gratitude, I offered a prayer to the One who answered my prayer back in my car, nine years before in Hollywood.

"Lord, thank you," I prayed. "I am very thankful to be in this place at this time, under this moon, alive and well. I don't have a great deal of money, and yet I feel wealthy. I have a disease that was supposed to take my life five years ago, and yet today I still feel healthy. I don't have much materially, Lord, but if I have enough faith to follow my heart and live out the dream you have given me, then surely I'm the wealthiest man I know. Thank you for my life, Lord. I'm happy to be here. I'm happy to be alive."

Just then, as if responding to my words, something slimy wriggled and slithered right under my feet. I was standing on top of some living thing! I jumped up and recoiled my feet. Looking down in the crystal clear moonlit water, I saw what at first appeared to be a white eel uncoiling itself where I had been standing. "An eel!" I thought excitedly. I had never seen an eel outside of an aquarium.

As the creature straightened itself out and began to swim past my knees, I decided to follow it. For a few feet I trailed after it, looking down, until I realized it wasn't an eel at all. It had the look of a snake. It was undoubtedly a white snake in the sea. What was a snake doing in the ocean? Terrified, I swam as fast as I could back to shore.

The next day in Morne Rouge I recounted to Marcel how the night before I had been standing on a snake in the sea. He pulled his cigar from his lips and his mouth dropped open.

"Adan," he asked in astonishment. "What color was that snake?"

Not understanding his expression, I described what I saw. "It was a white snake." Both Marcel and Gregory looked at each other in disbelief.

"That was a white sea snake, Adan! It is one of the

most poisonous snakes in the world," Marcel went on. "If that snake had bitten you, Adan, you wouldn't be here now to talk about it. Instead, you would be dead."

Mysterious are the ways of karma. Mysterious, indeed, is this life.

My disease has taken me much deeper into life than I ever would have gone without it. My disease has been my teacher, making me a better and truer human being. Though I would not wish it on another, and though I wish it might be otherwise for myself, my disease has been a gift to me nonetheless—a gift whose origin I believe is divine, and whose inner lessons I have yet to fully uncover.

Even so, certainly I know this much it has taught me: Wherever I go, I am my own home. As frail as my body may be, illness strengthens my spirit. Things are not as they seem on the surface, but as they are felt in the heart. God dwells within my heart as love, and my love for God is best expressed as gratitude.

Disease has taken me beyond the confines of this body, and I know without a shadow of a doubt that my self is the self of all. Embrace life, I say, no matter what it looks like, come what may. You never know what you will find just around the next corner.

Chapter Four

Interaction, Negotiation, and Relationships

We do not live apart from others. Healthy or not, we interact with family, friends, lovers, and strangers we encounter. Illness or disability can complicate our relationships. This chapter presents examples of interactions, which range from casual to intimate. We see how people's preconceived notions can disrupt our day-to-day lives. The writing reflects how we express ourselves within relationships and also shows how our loved ones can be affected.

What You See Ain't What You Get

Patricia Wellingham-Jones

I've been sliced and diced
and carved up nice,
put back together
with plastic and wire.
I sashay forth, head high,
chest out,
take on the world
I meet.
So, buddy, when the lights are low,
the mood's right, we're feeling tight,
I'll strip down to the skin
I live in.
You'd better get ready.
Brace your knees, stir that juice.
'Cause I'm me,
one hell of a woman,
and those knives
didn't change *me* at all.

Concentration

Erin Lewy

Jeremy's palm is rough under the pad of my thumb as I trace soft circles into his skin. My hand is shaking a little—his too—but I am not nervous. He takes a deep breath and smiles up at me. This is what he wants, and he's patient.

We laugh about things. The two of us are good at that—it's the best way to be. Earlier, during dinner, when the spasms in my hands were worse, I managed to get Parmesan cheese absolutely everywhere but into my bowl of pasta. Jeremy nearly dropped a forkful of linguini onto his lap but saved it at the last moment, well-practiced. "Gimp girl: minus one; gimp boy: one," we joked. Jeremy had suggested I lose two whole points, considering the mess I had made. I told him not to push his luck. Besides, it was my kitchen, which put me on clean-up duty by default. He really had no right to count it double unless he wanted to volunteer a hand.

It was all very creative. Throw some glue and Parmesan cheese on a canvas, add some music, a dancing gimp, and you could make it into a performance piece about the trials and tribulations of life on Social Security Income, what with all the food wasted with spasms and bad coordination.

"Fact," he said in the dramatic tone of a movie-trailer voice-over, "Every three minutes a tablespoon of grated

Parmesan cheese is unintentionally lost to the world as a result of the congenital affliction cerebral palsy. Show a special person you care. Your local theatre personnel will be taking your tax-deductible Parmesan donation following the show."

"God, you could almost convince me someone's tried that. Exactly like that," I said, laughing. His smile lit up his green eyes, and that's when I kissed him.

In bed, we move slowly. It is the measured slowness that we both share, the key to our togetherness. Our laughter sounds different—is different—now. It is the laughter of success, of pride. We are here now. We are moving together, slow and steady, getting it right. Perfect.

Sometimes, if we go too fast, the spasms happen. Jeremy doesn't want to laugh: This is sex, this is making love. It is serious and something we work hard for. Sometimes, when I think of all the work, I get so tired.

Long ago, I gave up asking social workers and doctors questions about sex. You can't ask questions. They look at you like you are a thing from Mars. They smile and pat your knee and say, "You've got such important things to worry about. Why this too? Are you even able to get around in this city? The other day I couldn't catch my train, even when I ran, and I thought of you. I think you ought to work on those kinds of problems." Their faces are a mix of disgust and pity. If only we weren't trapped in these horrid bodies, they could help us. They could support us in our quest for something more than a sufficient quantity of Ramen noodles, a special van, patient trains. But as it is—no, dear, no. Please don't make us think about that.

I prop myself up on one elbow and kiss Jeremy's sweet lips, running one hand through his hair. He swallows hard and closes his eyes. He is not afraid. He is concentrating. I run my fingers along the crease in the middle of his forehead, and he lets out his breath slowly, relaxes his concentration. His leg kicks out.

"Shit!" There is anger in his voice. "I could have kicked you," he says more quietly.

"That's okay," I say. "That's how you move. Besides, it's safer for you to kick me below the belt than it is for me to kick you there, so we're lucky." I smooth back his hair again. A smile is present, though reluctant, on his face. His eyes are wet. "Jer, this is me. I love you. It doesn't matter."

"I know. I know. I just hate it when I kick you. Jesus. I wouldn't give a shit about anything else—you know that. But I fucking hate it that I kick you."

"You'd do something else," I say matter-of-factly. "So let it go, babe." When I kiss him again, I am more insistent; it is deep and long and hot, and he forgets. He forgets the hate and he forgets the spasms and he kicks me, and we don't mind at all.

Jer and I know the movements of one another's bodies. This was not something we could rush into. Learning what works took a lot of waiting, watching. Before learning how to move together, we had to watch how we moved apart. We had to come to trust what we know and to trust each other. We had to learn to hold each other and make it count. Sex is huge and looming, and takes working up to. Before the big things can go smoothly, the smaller things need attention. Not that it has the tendency to go smoothly, even now. Smooth and easy sex is not Jeremy and me. We know this. It is not something we want, not really. And yet we get tired—tired of abortive attempts, of our bodies telling us "no" when we can hardly see straight from the want of it.

Quick and easy sex isn't really that great. Sure, it works, but where's the imagination? Jer knows I know the difference. When he's tired of it all, he reminds me of my time with Rob, who could walk, get on top, hold me without shaking. Then Jer is angry, hurt by his own thoughts. Sometimes, I can't say anything. When he is in this mood and won't listen, I do not want to touch him. I can't be a part of his negativity. I understand it; but in those moments it belongs to him, and he wants to keep it as such.

I think of Rob, the way he moved, the way things were then, how they worked. They were simpler, but not softer. Quicker, but not better. Less patient, more primal. More demanding. Rob moved my hands and legs where he thought they should go.

"Please," Jeremy says, "There. Please." He smiles. He waits. Helps me if I ask—if he can. And we don't mind.

Rob never waited. Never held me close and just lay there with me. He could move well and had to keep moving well, and so he moved me and then moved on.

I ask Jeremy, "Who's here with me now?" He says, "You think about him." Yes, I do. Sometimes, when I am at a loss for other words, I shout, "You're thinking about it, too!" Then he is quiet for a long time, and I know I have hurt him. We look down, then up, then move toward each other, smiling soft, apologetic smiles. We admit our pettiness, and we hold each other again.

With Jeremy, we speak softly and we move slowly; this

is our love. When I run my hands lightly over his body, he shivers. We claim each other with our hands, our tongues, fire spreading between us. We are together—only sight and sound and sensation. No fear, no hate, no pain. Only Jeremy and me. Together and moving slowly.

Somewhere a Mockingbird

Deborah Kent

When I was only a few weeks old, my mother realized that I couldn't see. For the next eight months, she and my father went from doctor to doctor searching for answers. At last, their quest led them to one of the leading eye specialists in New York City. He confirmed everything they had already heard by that time—my blindness was complete, irreversible, and of unknown origin. He also gave them some sound advice. They should stop taking me to doctors, give up looking for a cure. Instead, they should help me lead the fullest life possible. Fortunately for me, his prescription matched their best instincts.

As I was growing up, people called my parents "wonderful." They were praised for raising me "like a normal child." As far as I could tell, my parents were like most of the others in my neighborhood—sometimes wonderful and sometimes annoying. From my point of view, I wasn't LIKE a normal child, I WAS normal. From the beginning, I learned to deal with the world as a blind person. I didn't long for sight any more than I yearned for a pair of wings. Blindness presented occasional complications, but it seldom kept me from anything I wanted to do.

For me, blindness was part of the background music that accompanied my life. I had been hearing it since I was born and paid it little attention. But others had a way of cranking up the volume. Their discomfort, doubts, and concerns often put blindness at the top of the program. Teachers offered to lighten my assignments; Scout leaders discouraged me from going on field trips; boys shied away from asking me on dates. The message was clear. Because I was blind these people saw me as a liability—inadequate, incompetent, and too strange to be socially acceptable.

I knew that my parents ached for me when these situations arose. It hurt them to see me being prejudged and rejected. Yet they found it hard to do battle on my behalf. Though they shared my sense of injury, they also identified with the non-disabled people who sought to exclude me. "You have to understand how other people see things," my parents told me. "They're trying their best. You need to be patient with them." I struggled to show the doubters and detractors that they were wrong. Much of the time I felt that I was fighting alone.

Since one of my brothers is also blind, it seemed more than likely that my unknown eye condition had a genetic basis. I never thought much about it until my husband Dick and I began to talk about having a child. Certainly genetics was not our primary concern. We married late (I was 31, Dick 42) and were used to living unencumbered. Since we both worked as freelance writers, our income was erratic. We had to think about how we could shape our lives to make room for a child, whatever child that might be.

But somehow blindness crept into our discussions. I don't remember which of us brought up the topic first. But once it emerged, it had to be addressed. How would I feel if I passed my blindness to our son or daughter?

What would it mean to Dick and to our extended families? What would it be like for us to raise a blind child together? I premised my life on the conviction that blindness was a neutral characteristic. It created some inconveniences, such as not being able to read print or drive a car. Occasionally it locked me into conflicts with others over what I could and could not do. But in the long run I believed that my life could not have turned out any better if I had been fully sighted. If my child were blind, I would try to ensure it every chance to become a self-fulfilled, contributing member of society. Dick said he agreed with me completely. We were deciding whether to have a child. Its visual acuity was hardly the point.

Yet if we believed our own words, why were we discussing blindness at all? I sensed that Dick was trying hard to say the right thing, even to believe it in his heart. But he was more troubled than he wished me to know. Once, when I asked him how he would feel if he learned that our child was blind, he replied, "I'd be devastated at first, but I'd get over it." It was not the answer I wanted to hear.

I was blind and I was the woman Dick chose to marry, to spend his life with for better or for worse. I was his partner in all our endeavors. He accepted my blindness naturally and comfortably, as a piece of who I was. If he could accept blindness in me, why would it be devastating to him, even for a moment, if our child were blind as well? "You know why," was all he could tell me. "You've got to understand."

What I understood was that Dick, like my parents, was the product of a society that views blindness, and all disability, as fundamentally undesirable. All his life he had been assailed by images of blind people who were helpless, useless, and unattractive, misfits in a sight-oriented world. I had managed to live down that image. Dick had discovered that I had something of value to offer. But I had failed to convince him that it is really okay to be blind.

Our discussions showed me a painful truth. No matter how close we grew, how much of our lives we shared, blindness would never be a neutral trait for him. I wanted our child to be welcomed without reservation. I wanted Dick to greet its birth with joy. I did not know if I could bear his devastation if our baby turned out to be blind like me.

It was too painful to explore the implications any further. Instead, I plunged into a search for information. After all, we didn't even know the real cause of my blindness. We couldn't make a decision until we gathered the facts. Surely the field of ophthalmology had learned something new over the past three decades. A series of phone calls led me to a specialist at New York University Medical Center. I was assured that if anyone could answer my questions, he was the man.

On a sunny morning in October, Dick and I set out for New York to learn why I am blind. We lived in a small town in central Pennsylvania at the time, and Dick wasn't used to driving in the city. He dreaded the horn-blaring, bumper-to-bumper traffic and the desperate search for a parking space. All of his energy focused on delivering us to our destination. As we packed the car he commented, "It's going to be a long, nervous day." I couldn't have agreed with him more.

Parking on the streets of Manhattan was as difficult

as Dick had feared. Finally, we squeezed into a spot a dozen blocks from the hospital and set out on foot. The city engulfed us with its fumes and bustle and grinding noise. We didn't try to talk above the traffic. There was nothing new to say.

We had walked several blocks when I was dimly aware of a strange sound. It was remarkably like the song of a bird—the clear, warbling notes ringing out against the concrete walls around us. At first I assumed it was a recording turned full blast or some mechanical toy worked by a child. But as we drew nearer Dick remarked, "There's a crowd of people standing by a tree. They're all looking at something. Oh hey, there's a bird up there!"

I've been an avid birder most of my life, and the song was unmistakable. It was a mockingbird. The mockingbird thrives in fields and gardens. It gathers scraps and snippets from the songs of other birds and braids them into a pattern all its own. The mockingbird sings exuberantly from April to June, but by late summer it usually falls silent. Yet this one poured forth its song on East 32nd Street in mid October, out of place and out of season. It seemed utterly fearless and confident, staking a claim for itself in that inhospitable city landscape. It had something to say, and it was determined to be heard.

New Yorkers are used to almost anything, but the extraordinary song of this tiny creature brought them to a standstill. For a little while Dick and I paused too. We stood on the pavement, listening and marveling. Then we pushed through the revolving door and into the antiseptic halls of the medical center.

I expected a battery of tests, maybe a referral to yet another expert. But the doctor dilated my pupils, gazed into my eyes, and announced, “I’ll tell you what you have, and I’m 100 percent certain. You’ve got Leber’s congenital amaurosis.” Leber’s is a genetic condition, he explained, autosomal recessive in nature. Both of my parents carried the recessive gene, and each of their children had a one-in-four chance of inheriting the eye condition. What were my chances of passing Leber’s on to my own children, I asked. The doctor explained that I would inevitably give one recessive gene for Leber’s to my child. But unless my partner happened to carry the same recessive gene, there was no possibility that our child would be affected. The chances were slight that Dick would prove to be another carrier.

The discussion could have ended with that simple exchange of information. But the doctor had more to say. “You have a good life, don’t you?” he asked. “If you have a child with Leber’s, it can have a good life, too. Go home and have a dozen kids if you want to!”

Even from a total stranger those were wonderful words. They affirmed that I was not a liability to the world. I was a worthwhile human being with a variety of traits to pass on to future generations. To this New York doctor my Leber’s genes were not a curse. They need not be extinguished any more than my genes for dark-brown hair. I was valued for who I was. My child, sighted or blind, could be valued in the same way. I floated out of the doctor’s office and found Dick in the packed waiting room.

“Hey, guess what!” I cried in triumph. “I’ve got Leber’s congenital amaurosis!”

The trip to New York cemented our decision to have a child. We left the city with a new certainty, a sense that we were ready for whatever came our way. Yet I knew Dick was comforted by the fact that Leber's is relatively rare and that probably he did not carry the recessive gene. I wished that he didn't need that comfort.

Within the year we were parents-to-be. We awaited the birth of our child with all the eagerness, wonder, and anxiety common to expectant parents. We seldom mentioned the possibility that our baby might be blind. Leber's congenital amaurosis seemed safely remote, a flash of lightning that wouldn't strike again. But it could reappear, I knew. I lived with the small, unspoken fear that if our child were blind, Dick would feel betrayed—by medical science, by fate, by me.

Dick had his doubts about coaching me through labor and viewing the birth. To support us both, his sister came along to our Lamaze classes. She stayed with us in the birthing room to help out in case Dick should faint dead away. But nobody fainted. When our daughter Janna arrived we greeted her with greater joy than I could have imagined. Her welcome was boundless and wholly unreserved.

My parents flew out to visit us when we brought Janna home from the hospital. Mom helped with the cooking and housecleaning and insisted that I get as much rest as I could. I spent every conscious moment nursing, rocking, diapering, and marveling at the extraordinary new being who had entered our lives. I was too happy and excited to feel exhaustion.

I wasn't worried about Janna's vision or anything else. But one day my mother confided that my father had told her, "We've still got to find out if the baby's blind." I was stunned by his concern and by her unquestioning acceptance that it was justified. My parents raised all three of their children, including my blind brother and me, with sensitivity and unwavering love. In all of us they tried to nurture confidence, ambition, and self-respect. Yet they felt apprehensive about the prospect that their granddaughter might also be blind. Blindness had never become neutral for them, any more than it had for Dick.

It was almost time for Mom and Dad to go home when Dick said to my mother, "You've raised two blind children. What do you think? Can this kid see or not?" My mother said she really couldn't be sure. Janna was barely a week old. It was too soon to tell. The day after my parents left, Dick found the answer on his own. As Janna lay in his arms, awake and alert, he moved his hand back and forth above her face. Distinctly, he saw her turn her head to track the motion. She saw his hand. She followed it with her eyes.

"She can see!" Dick exulted. He rushed to the phone and called my parents with the news. I listened quietly to their celebrations. I don't know if anyone noticed that I had very little to say.

How do I feel about the fact that Janna can see? I am glad that her world is enriched by color as well as texture and sound. When she snaps a picture with her new camera or poses before the mirror in her favorite dress I draw pleasure from her delight. As her mother, I want her to have every advantage, and I know that some aspects of her life are easier because she has sight. She can play video games with her friends; she can thumb through magazines and note the latest fashions. All too soon now she will be learning to drive a car.

Beyond that, I am glad Janna will never be dismissed

as incompetent and unworthy simply because she is blind. I am grateful that she will not face the discrimination that threads its way through my life and the lives of most people with disabilities. But I know her vision will not spare her from heartbreak. She will still meet disappointment, rejection, and self-doubt, as all of us must.

I will always believe that blindness is a neutral trait, neither to be prized nor shunned. Very few people, not even those dearest to me, share that conviction. My husband, my parents, and so many others who are central to my life cannot fully relinquish their negative assumptions. I feel that I have failed when I run into jarring reminders that I have not changed their perspective. In those crushing moments I fear that I am not truly accepted after all.

But in recent years a new insight has gradually come to me. Yes, my own loved ones hold the unshakeable belief that blindness is and always will be a problem. Nevertheless, these same people have made me welcome. Though they dread blindness as a fate to be avoided at almost any cost, they give me their trust and respect. I don't understand how they live without discomfort amid such contradictions. But I recognize that people can and do reach out, past centuries of prejudice and fear, to forge bonds of love. It is a truth to marvel at, a cause for hope and perhaps some small rejoicing.

Sometimes Dick reminisces about the day Janna turned her head to watch his moving fingers. In his voice I hear an echo of the excitement and relief that were so vivid for him on that long-ago morning. Each time I hear the story I feel a twinge of the old pain, and for a few moments I am very much alone again.

But I have my own favorite stories to recall. I remember our long, nervous day in New York and the doctor who told me to go home and have a dozen kids. And somehow I have never forgotten the mockingbird that sang so boldly in a place where no one thought it belonged, making a crowd of busy people stand still to listen.

The Wig

Hugh Burns, O.P.

"Just get a piece." This was the advice I received from a sympathetic friend. He even offered to pay for it. We would go to the salon of the wigmaker to the stars, who would provide me with the very best in artificial hirsutude. My beneficent friend had just confronted the new me—my head naked and smooth. From the back I could have filled in for a ripe honeydew melon at the farmers' market. Since that day, he has renewed his generous offer annually, which I also graciously decline each year.

That was sixteen years ago. I had come down with alopecia universalis, an autoimmune disorder that causes hair loss. In my case, with an immune system locked in overdrive, I was left as completely plucked as a fully dressed Thanksgiving turkey. Thus, the universalis—complete hair loss—the full nine yards or at least all five feet ten inches of me.

Physically this condition has no other deleterious side effects. As it kills off the hair follicles, however, it also rips up one's emotional stability and sense of identity. The head is, after all, one's most salient characteristic. In a matter of two short weeks I was rendered unrecognizable to friends, family, and colleagues. I didn't even know the guy in my bathroom mirror anymore.

Soon after the diagnosis I took a trip to Chile. Those were still the days of General Pinochet and I was detained in the Santiago airport. The immigration officer examining my documents had won the Heinrich Himmler look alike contest in his full-length black leather coat and high peaked SS cap. It took several hours to convince him that this hairless gringo was the same person as the fully-fledged man in the passport picture.

From the beginning I opted against any kind of treatment. None of the prescribed salves, hormones, or steroids offered much hope in a case as extreme as mine anyway. A well meaning Guatemalan housekeeper promised that a paste made of sweet potatoes and sulphur would sprout a new crop within a week. My dermatologist wanted to shoot needles full of cortisone into my skull to stimulate growth. I waved him off. "At least let me bring back your eyebrows," he pleaded. As the cortisone would eventually collapse my forehead muscles, he advised pumping in enough silicone to keep me from looking like a face-lift headed for a malpractice suit. Thanks but no thanks.

After attending several support meetings for alopecia, I also decided against a wig. At one meeting, a high-powered Washington lawyer revealed how his alopecia had devastated both his personal and professional lives. Now under the therapeutic cover of a hairpiece he testified to a new found self-confidence. He could face the world as a normal person again. Sure I could empathize, but the thing looked like a football helmet. Good or bad, human hair or dynel, a toupee was not for me. Overall it was just a lot easier to accept the new me. Besides, in recent years my dome has become a "look" both stylish and sexy. Trent Lott and Congressman Trafficant, eat your hearts out!

I thought I had resolved the matter of a wig long ago, but last year my big-hearted, piece-pushing friend duped me. He needed a ride to his renowned wigmaker to the stars. His own "toup" was due for a tune-up. It was time to add more silver strands to match the graying sidewalls around his ears. All this only made me more grateful I had long ago chosen to go au naturel. Naively I suspected nothing.

We pulled up to a nondescript professional building. Among the various notations on the directory for physicians, dentists, and accountants, there was one for "Hair Replacement Studio." How discreet and understated, I thought. Upon opening the door all discretion was annihilated.

We stood at the threshold of a crowded waiting room. The chic furnishings were complemented by ubiquitous, poster-sized photos of smartly bewigged men. The décor stood in stark contrast to the clients huddled around the reception area. They were all men in various stages of baldness or the camouflaging thereof. None of them looked happy. The scene reminded me of the emergency room at St. Vincent's Hospital on a rough Saturday night. After the door opened they glanced around furtively, hoping that no one they knew had walked through.

My eye was immediately drawn to three cast-down heads, each draped in a washcloth. They were obviously in the midst of some several staged process of treatment—ugly ducklings indeed, awaiting their full plumage. They resembled forlorn models bumped from a Vermeer sitting. Somehow I couldn't picture Burt Reynolds or William Shatner sitting around under a towel in this waiting room for the wigmaker to the stars.

A feeling of immediate unease washed over me. No way would I submit myself to the humiliation of sitting there on display, by the door no less, under a napkin with whatever epoxy or fertilizer it was incubating.

Before I could absorb the whole scene, both my friend and I were deftly whisked into an elegantly appointed cubicle. The door shut softly but resolutely. Suddenly I was unwittingly sitting in a sleek salon chair staring at myself in the mirror. The wigmaker to the stars himself, no mere assistant, was standing behind me—with a full head of his own hair and not one of his fabulous creations, I might add. His hands were firmly clamped down on my shoulders. I wasn't going anywhere.

Like Dorothy waking up in Oz, I wondered how I ended up in that chair. Slinking down into a fetal position, I felt like a toddler awaiting the unknown of his first haircut. "There must be some mistake," I protested. "I'm only the chauffeur for the other gentleman who wanted a few gray hairs sewn into his own piece. Thanks, but I'll just wait outside." I was captive. There was no convincing anyone in that kangaroo court that they had the wrong guy. I was an undocumented alien in this hair replacement cell, where my rights as a free agent no longer applied. My increasingly adamant protests fell on increasingly deaf ears.

From a drawer the wigmaker produced a large ring, like a jailer's, festooned with tufts of hair samples in every imaginable tint. Blond was chosen for me. It would look more natural I was assured with unflinching confidence. For a more realistic look I was advised to add some gray, given my age. "Oh no," I declared, "there wasn't any gray when it fell out and there won't be any when it goes back on." That was non-negotiable. These new guardians of my vanity were beaming at my expression of such resolution. Very well, ageless blond it would be. Just as I wished. They were smiling in sweet unison at my tacit submission to their custody.

It was obvious that I was now a co-conspirator in this reforestation project. It was no longer a question of whether to start planting, but what kind of foliage would look best. The choice was all mine, the unctuous voice of the wigmaker sighed. But first the piece had to be handcrafted. Then I would come in for the final styling and shaping. Amidst my futile protests, tape measures were wound around my cranium. All this geometry, no doubt divided by pi, was delivered to the weavers in the back room. I was well on my way to becoming someone else. Having adjusted to myself as Kojack, I was going to be a Beach Boy.

Just to get an idea of what it might look like, an unstyled, off-the-rack mop was dropped onto my head. Under this canopy of tousled, sand colored locks, I looked like Ringo Starr on the Ed Sullivan Show. Once it was styled, I was assured no one would know I was wearing a piece—only the discreet wigmaker and my not so discreet, conniving friend.

And because I was such a sport, and my friend no doubt such a loyal and frequent buyer, the wigmaker's wife was going to throw in a bonus pair of eyebrows. She appeared and produced two fuzzy strips along with a bottle of glue. They sat in her palm like a couple of caterpillars.

I noticed that the wife was Spanish speaking. I pleaded with her in my most elegant and forceful Castilian:

"Yo no las quiero!" I had expected more sympathy for victim's rights from the opposite sex. No such luck. With one artful sweep of her dainty hands, she slapped those two strips across my naked brow. They were perfectly sculpted and shaped and better suited to Mrs. Doubtfire or Dustin Hoffman's "Tootsie."

The three of them stood around me like Job's compatriots. They countered every one of my objections with the assurance that I would be happy once I finally had my hair back—or someone else's. Besides the whole thing was paid for. And not to worry, my flahoolagh friend had already arranged to cover all future styling, shaping, washing, setting, tinting, or whatever fancy I fancied—in perpetuity. What a sweetheart deal, win win all around. Why wasn't I convinced?

As we left the salon I pretended not to be a defeated man. With one breath I was still protesting. With the next I was asking about which coiffure was for me. My friend looked pleased as my tone shifted from resolute negative to an ambiguity he perceived morphing into blessed resignation. He eased the transition with a couple of Cuba libres over an ocean-view lunch. There was no use in fighting it. With age my face might sag and shrivel, but that wig would remain defiantly and forever blond. I would be Robert Redford-usque ad mortem.

It's just a hat. That was my friend's mantra. Like subliminal suggestion, he was convinced that if he repeated it enough it would bring me around. He advised that I could always pull a Willard Scott and swing both ways—go with or without at whim. In addition the piece would allow me to go incognito. I replied that I actually thrilled at being recognized. And besides if I was doing something I didn't want to be recognized at, I probably shouldn't be doing it. Or at least I wouldn't want to be doing it with a prosthesis precariously matted down on my scalp.

The more we talked about the details of the care of this new accessory, the more I realized this was not just another Yankees cap. It could be rinsed out in the sink, blow- dried or just hung up in the shower. And then there were the pros and cons of the various shampoos and conditioners. Or I could just take up my friend's generous offer and send it back to the wigmaker from anywhere in the world for refurbishing. My unadorned head was spinning. I had been free of all tonsorial concerns for the last sixteen years. Just a hat? This thing was more like a pet.

"God only made a few perfect heads and the rest He put hair on." If I had a quarter for every time in the last sixteen years someone has come up to me with that stale line, I'd be driving a BMW. Rather than tell them where they might deposit their dated joke book, I just dredge up a phony belly laugh and act as if I had never heard it before. But that afternoon at that little, old wigmaker's, I suddenly realized that I did have one of those perfect heads. No dents or bumps, no age spots or scars. I didn't have a Gorbachev blotch the shape of Antarctica on top of my world. And now they were going to cover it all up! This was a crime against art, like tacking down indoor/ outdoor carpet on a parquet oak floor.

OK, maybe I do miss the hair at the beach. It is, after all, nature's sunscreen for at least one body part. But a wig at the beach? In a pounding surf? One's pride and dignity, and not to mention hefty investment, are in definite peril. I don't care how good that glue is.

I arrived back home awash in a whirlpool of emotions. I was confused, depressed, distraught, angry. Mostly I was mad at myself. I had allowed myself to be hoodwinked. Wait a minute, I am the bald guy. I wouldn't know how to be any other way. And I like me the way I am.

I decided to call and cancel. I still had time. Only four hours had passed. It was a quarter to six and there were fifteen minutes before closing. Taking back my independence, I punched out the number on the telephone keys as if they were the wigmaker's lights. Identifying myself to the receptionist I boldly asserted: "Cancel the order, please!"

It was too late. The wig was already being hand-sewn. With all his clout and schmoozing of the wigmaker, my friend had put a top priority, extra urgent rush on the thing. I could just picture the scene of its manufacture: a dimly lit sweatshop crammed with a boatload of Haitian women chained to their workbenches. They were feverishly stitching individual golden strands by the millions onto the fine mesh of my cranial measurements, slaving 15-hour days, deprived of bathroom breaks and making fifty cents an hour. Several more reasons to cancel it.

No one, not even the wigmaker to the stars, could halt the process now. The stern voice at the other end, with a tone of reprimand, informed me that my change of mind would require a personal conversation with the wigmaker himself. It sounded as if I was to be given a penance for my capriciousness. But alas, the wigmaker was out of town for a few days. By the time he returned, the piece would be finished. "He sure cleared out quickly and conveniently enough," I said under my breath.

I suggested that they donate it to a needy chemotherapy patient. Not possible. This piece was custom made for me and like Cinderella's slipper it would fit no one else. Well cancellation or not, I informed her, I would not be making such a phone call to the wigmaker and I would not be by to pick it up—ever!

The next day I called my friend to ease whatever strain my assertiveness had placed on our relationship. He confessed that he felt badly too for pushing the toupee on me. We apologized back and forth like a pair of Geisha girls bowing in incessant, alternating rhythm. No matter, he already knew about my cancellation. The wigmaker had called him. It crossed my mind that the guy lost no time, from whatever retreat he had spirited himself off to, to respond to my challenge. Our exchange of antiphonal mea culpas ended with my friend reminding me that nonetheless my blond piece was paid for. It would always be in a box in his dresser drawer, in case I ever had a change of heart. He sheepishly added, "But how about those stick-on eyebrows?"

The Energy Monster

Laban Carrick Hill

My seven-year-old daughter Natalie calls it "The Energy Monster." Natalie drew a picture of it on a large piece of paper in the office of our family therapist. In the drawing the Energy Monster stands at the foot of my bedroom. This monster has big teeth, angry eyes, and either a jagged black tongue or a very strange, expressively-shaped text balloon coming out of its mouth. The monster is orange with hair cut short like mine. Encircled by orange loop-de-loops, it is in a "frenzy."

In the picture I am brown and am lying on a yellow bed, my head on a pillow. I'm covered by a brown blanket that has been cross-sectioned like one of those children's science or "howthings-work" books that show the inside and outside simultaneously. The blanket is pulled up to my chin, but the side of the blanket has not been drawn in, so my left side is exposed. She has drawn a shirt, pants, and shoes on me in a nod toward modesty since in truth I wear only boxer shorts to bed. Whether it is her modesty or mine she is preserving is unclear.

I am in obvious danger. The monster could pounce on me at any moment while I lie prone on the yellow bed—no chance to defend myself.

Tucked under one foot of the energy monster and drawn in red marker is a building that could be our house if our house were a three-story building instead of a ranch. Some of the orange-lined frenzy of the Energy Monster overlaps the outline of the building.

Incongruously, Natalie has scribbled a bright yellow sun in the upper right hand corner of the page. In red marker she has placed herself and her younger sister Ella cramped in the lower left hand corner beside the house. She stands there smiling while Ella has no face. In all of Natalie's pictures she is smiling. I have always found this fact pleasing because I imagine this suggests she has a positive self view.

As I examine the picture more closely, I notice that Natalie is actually closer to the Energy Monster than I am. I ask her why she did that.

She points to a black line she has drawn separating the monster from her and Ella. "There wasn't enough room," she answers. "So I drew this line to separate us."

Then, I ask her what is she doing.

She says she is waiting.

Waiting for what? I press.

She tells me she is waiting for the right moment to send the Energy Monster to California.

Why California?

Because there it will melt, she tells me.

I agree that California seems the most likely place for the Energy Monster to go since we live on the other side of the continent in Vermont.

Then, I look at the sun in the upper right hand corner and think it's not so inexplicable after all. I soak up the warmth of that bright yellow sun, drawn in an imperfect circle. I feel safe in its presence and let its imaginary rays restore the energy that the monster has stolen.

Natalie and I know the Energy Monster from different

points of view. She knows the beast as a creature that takes her father away from her and leaves an irritable, sad person. For me, the monster is a metaphor for my depression.

When the Energy Monster is here, I can't tell you why it has come or what route it has taken to get here. I am only conscious of its presence. I am depressed and can see no way out.

When people see me, I am told that I look listless, worn out, exhausted. My appearance is ragged. I stop shaving and brushing my teeth. I will wear the same shirt and pants for days on end. I prefer the dark and resist leaving the house, especially during the day. One summer two years ago, I didn't voluntarily leave the house for two months. During that time, I didn't mow the lawn or attend to any yard chores.

I can easily sleep sixteen, twenty hours a day. Oftentimes I will get up in the morning to help prepare Ella for preschool and Natalie for school. Then I will drive one or both to school. At this point my wife Elise goes to work while I return home and to bed, only to rise when it comes time to pick up the kids at the end of their day. Then I put the kids in front of the television to watch a video, and I prepare dinner. After supper I return to bed while Elise bathes the kids and gets them ready for bed. Once this is done, I read bedtime stories to one of my kids. Then I return to bed.

Combined with my enormous weariness is an insatiable hunger. When I am not sleeping, I am planning my next meal or eating it. I can eat so much it becomes nearly impossible to distinguish when one meal ends and another begins. If I must travel from one place to another, my route inevitably detours through the drive-up window of a fast food restaurant.

My therapist tells me that studies have shown that depressed people crave carbohydrates. The sugar into which the carbs convert offers a form of self-medication. The body somehow knows the person is depressed and so signals that it needs more bread, grains, potatoes, and other carbohydrates. The difficulty arises in that I do not turn to a twelve-grain bread sandwich packed with roasted vegetables and sprouts, but instead gravitate toward the foods I found comforting as a child—hamburgers, French fries, grilled cheese, salami submarines.

I think of this kind of eating as grazing. I imagine myself as livestock working my way across a meadow. At other times, I remember that my grandfather told me how horses drink water until their bellies explode. I'll look down at my bloated stomach and fear something like that can happen to me. I have no clear answer, but more importantly, I wouldn't stop even were the answer there.

When I'm awake, whether eating or not, I am reading. I lose myself in pulp fiction. This violent, paranoid, conspiratorial world somehow soothes the discomfort in my bones. I'm attracted to blunt, vicious, and unyielding darkness as characterized in the cover blurb of Jim Thompson's *The Alcoholics* (Berkley: Black Lizard Books, 1986):

> Murder wouldn't matter now, not after his brain was already dead. He'd be better off in the ground, anywhere but where he was, strapped to a table—a mute, tortured imbecile.

Or the first paragraph of Stephen Hunter's *Dirty White Boys* (NY: Random House, 1994):

> Three men at McAlester State Prison had larger penises than Lamar Pye, but all were black and therefore, by Lamar's own figuring, hardly human at all. His was the largest penis ever seen on a white man in that prison or any others in which Lamar had spent so much of his adult life. It was a monster, a snake, a ropey, veiny thing that hardly looked at all like what it is but rather like some form of rubber tubing.

The improbably raw and mean-spirited plots reinforce my sense that there is real danger and malice in my surrounding environment. I begin not simply to suspect, but to be actually convinced, that those around me wish me ill, that my family and friends do not like me, that they resent me. During one difficult period, I got it into my head that I could only drink from a glass that contained four ice cubes. Somehow I had reasoned that the proportion of ice to liquid in any sized glass was ideal with four ice cubes. It didn't seem to matter what size the ice cubes were—or how much liquid was poured into the glass. I was just focused on the four ice cubes. Whenever Elise did me the favor of offering to get me a drink, she would inevitably forget my rigid four-ice-cube dictum. She would put two or three or even five ice cubes in my glass. While I can now admit that I had neglected to remind her of my beverage policy, in the moment I would become inflamed and would then accuse her of trying to displace the exquisite balance I had achieved in my environment.

Simultaneously, I am certain that I have harmed my

family in some deeply important way and so deserve their abandonment. As I sit here at my desk, I can tell you these thoughts are as absurd as you might think. Of course, I know that they aren't true, and even when I'm depressed there's a part of me that knows this. Still, it feels that way. And through some weird alchemy that I'm still untangling, in this state feelings are facts.

It used to be that I believed the Energy Monster to be supernatural. That it followed laws beyond nature. That was why the Energy Monster could descend upon me out of the blue. It was as if I really did wake up on the wrong side of the bed, but all four sides were wrong. Then, just as miraculously, the beast would vanish in a cloud of mystery.

With the work I've done in hospital programs and intensive therapy, and the new kinds of medications available for clinically depressed people, I've come to understand that this is not the case. The monster is anchored in very real biological and psychological circumstances. The most effective treatment I've had has been in what is called a partial hospitalization program that I would attend from 9 a.m. to 4 p.m. each day. This program was organized around the tenets of Cognitive Behavioral Therapy. I attended the program twice over the course of a year. The focus of my work there was to identify and become conscious of habits of thinking that would distort my reading of situations. I learned how these cognitive distortions prepared me for and then propelled me into depression. My therapist and I have continued to work on these techniques, and I have seen real progress in my ability to function and, even, enjoy life.

Nevertheless, this new understanding is not a cure-all. In this way I am not like many who get situationally depressed or experience a period of depression in their lives and fully recover. I think of my friend Susan who suffered depression for many years, but has recovered without a relapse with the help of Zoloft. I look at Elise who recently lost her job. This event sent her into a deep depression, which lasted several weeks. Her feelings passed eventually—however. They were situational. When the situation changed, the depression lifted.

That my depression does not follow one of these patterns has caused me much distress over the years. In fact, for my entire life. As a child I used to sit in church and listen to people testify about one affliction or another. They would describe how their faith in the Lord and prayer had lifted their need for alcohol or their lustings after another's wife or husband. Then, we would sing a hymn that underscored how they were lost and now they were found by the Lord. As I listened to these miracles, I'd wish that it could happen to me. Then I would pray for my pain to be lifted as well, but it never happened. For years I wondered if I were bad or evil in some way I couldn't identify because I could not be saved.

I felt my affliction was more primal. Its roots were not in the New Testament, but rather in ancient mythology. I was damned much like Sisyphus who was forced to roll a boulder up one of two hills, and each time he reached the top, the boulder would roll back down and Sisyphus would have to start anew. In my worst moments, I imagined myself allied with Prometheus who was chained to a rock, where his liver was eaten daily by a vulture, and grew back nightly, only to be eaten again the following day.

At times, I still characterize my depression in epic proportions, but Natalie's drawing has tempered this inflation of feeling. It shows me the "cartoonish" texture of my dramas. Like a slasher movie, all of these narratives are from the victim's point of view where the monster is some hideous, unknown entity that is out to do me harm.

For this reason, I keep the picture tacked on the bulletin board in my office. When I talk on the phone or pause for a moment, my eyes rest on the drawing. As I look at it now, I'm reminded of what I've learned.

This beast has very distinct and recognizable travel plans. The Energy Monster never simply arrives unannounced. Instead, I can see it books its flight from California well in advance. This Monster is frugal. It wants the best package it can get—meaning it wants me to pay as dear a price as can be extracted.

The Energy Monster will start packing its bags whenever I begin to feel isolated. If Elise and I have an argument or disagreement that is not easily resolvable, I can feel my anxiety level increase. The first signs might be that I dream that night of losing her in some catastrophic way—a car accident, an earthquake, cancer. The first ten years of my marriage I would do anything not to come into conflict with Elise. I used to brag to my friends that Elise and I never fought. I can see this pathology now as my unconscious effort to thwart the Energy Monster. It's a simple syllogism: if Elise and I don't fight, I won't be anxious. Therefore, I won't become depressed.

Over the years, I went to great lengths to keep myself out of situations that held potential conflict. I used to joke that I lived by the Boy Scout Code: Safety First. My sensory perceptions became finely tuned for any static in my environment. At a magazine job I had when I was in my early twenties, my boss was particularly irascible. Before I took the position to be his assistant, he had gone through three people in six months.

In some ways I view that job experience as my training ground. I learned to be very skilled at modulating his moods. Elise, who worked for the same magazine, used to joke that everyone thought I was on Valium because I handled him so well. In truth, I was so calm because I was exhausted. All my attention was focused on keeping this man happy. When he was upset or angry, I would find some way to change his mood. I might go out and buy him ice cream. Or I might share a particularly delicious piece of office gossip. Usually, I simply acted like a devoted puppy. When he was in a good mood, I worked hard to protect it. I would deflect all bad news. I would hold potentially combustive phone messages aside until I could find a safe way to pass them along.

In that small office we shared at the end of a hall, I learned to be an exquisite listening device. Much like the seismometer that geologists use, I was an instrument that received and measured the environmental conditions for conflict. Often, I could do this long distance over the phone. Sometimes, I'd use this skill like a psychic to predict potential conflict that lay in the future. Then, I would strenuously avoid those situations. I can remember at the time never wanting to be in the same room with two friends who did not like each other. I couldn't tolerate their enmity even though their dislike had nothing to do with me. Deep down, I felt that I was not only responsible for their conflict, but also responsible for resolving something that could not be resolved by me. The only logical response then was simply to avoid their company.

As it was bound to, this exquisite instrument failed. As I grew older, I had to modify it repeatedly until it was more like a Rube Goldberg contraption than the instrument I had originally constructed. I developed such sensitivity to any shift in environmental conditions that I became immobilized. The infinitesimal nuances and shifts of emotional energy in a room were too complex to process and then to form into an appropriate response.

As I lie in bed, the Energy Monster threatening me has come to represent this condition so clearly. I am enormously grateful to Natalie for her inspired drawing. It has given me a starting point from which to trace the monster's journey backward. I can see now that it begins as a ticket of doubt in need of a customer. I then cash the doubt in with an experience, such as an ambiguous response from a friend that might leave me feeling unsettled. Like everyone, I sometimes invite a friend for dinner or to go to a movie and that friend can't do it. The next time I call with an invitation, that friend might be busy that night as well for any number of legitimate reasons. Without prompting, however, I'll find a way to blame myself and characterize the decline as cold rejection. With a sense of desperation I'll sort through my memory of the most recent encounters with this friend and identify numerous instances where I "probably" offended him. The consequences of my offending behavior have only one conclusion: As a result of my utter repulsiveness, my friend no longer wants to get together. The reasons are clearly self-evident.

My choice of career as a writer has offered a unique opportunity to cash in on this doubt as well. Often, when I mail a manuscript to an editor, I do not hear from them for months. Instead of calling to check on the editor's progress through my work, I create worst case scenarios: the editor is much too embarrassed or repulsed by the amateurishness, or the bald stupidity, of my efforts to feel it deserves a response. Ka-ching! The ticket has been purchased at full fare.

At this point the monster is ready to travel. It approaches slowly. At first it's a speck on the horizon. As I accumulate more experiences that reinforce my sense of inadequacy, the monster nears. It is as if the monster is now in a car, or a bus, traveling along a winding road and gaining speed with each pang of doubt. With the monster approaching, I can feel my tentative hold on my own sense of adequacy, even legitimacy, begin to loosen. Here, the monster picks up speed. He aims for my unprotected confidence and flattens it on the pavement. I survive, if it can be called survival, with only that wretched, yet intractable, organ of the spirit, worthlessness.

Out of this diminished state, my feelings of hopelessness emerge. Effortlessly, I globalize even further and conclude: whatever hopes I might have for my life are foolish, delusional. My being can then be reduced to a neat syllogism. I am unloved and unlovable. Therefore, I cannot exist. This simple logic would have sent Descartes to the asylum. These thoughts are mine. Therefore, I cannot exist.

* * *

Today, I think about tolerating a certain level of discomfort. I do this by operating at a deliberate pace that allows me to name and acknowledge my feelings as they arise. That way these feelings cannot spiral out of control unnoticed. One trick has been to avoid multitasking because trying to juggle several things at once distracts me from what I am feeling. Then these unrecognized feelings can easily transform into thoughts of disaster. I remind myself, instead, to stay connected with myself and others. I try to touch Elise a couple of times a day. Putting my hand on her shoulder or giving her a hug reminds me that I am loved. At the same time I've found exercise essential to my well-being. When I am conscious of my breath and the movement of my body, I feel physically stronger, and from this actual strength I sense myself as more capable of managing what lies beyond.

I joke with Elise that the Energy Monster has bought a condo in California. He's setting down roots there and won't want to come back. As I spin this narrative, I shift the paradigm of being Depression's victim just a little. My encounter with the monster I now view from its perspective as well as my own. He has a real home and real needs. Much like the monster in Mary Shelley's *Frankenstein*, my monster is normalized through this process. It no longer resides within the traditional horror story model—me a victim of its possession. Instead, I have come to see my circumstances from the monster's perspective, where I can discover the kind of sustenance it needs to survive alone in California.

I've come to learn much about my monster and our consanguinity. My daughter's drawing keeps me alert to discovering more about him so that some day, in the future, I can have the presence of mind to know when my feelings are myth—belonging therefore to the Monster—and when they are "mine." I must do this because what I've read about depression and what I've been told by my psychiatrist and my therapist is that the likelihood of the monster returning is high. I am not like my friend Susan or my wife Elise, or even the parishioners of my childhood. I cannot be relieved of its presence for eternity. I can just hope that the intervals between its return are longer and that its stays are shorter and less intense. I just hope . . . I can only hope.

The Café Lady

Raymond J. Aguilera

A few weeks ago I was sitting at my desk at work when a coworker asked me to join her for a cup of coffee. Desperately in need of a break, I agreed. We strolled down Telegraph Avenue and ducked into a café. Given that both of our respective love lives were in states of flux, I settled into my chair looking forward to some juicy gossip.

I should mention that my friend Alana uses an electric wheelchair with a ventilator strapped to the back. Anywhere else in the world she might be a remarkable sight, but cruising the streets of Berkeley, California, she appears remarkably ordinary. That simple fact, that a gimp like me and his big-ass-chair-drivin' friend can walk down the street without attracting much attention, is one of the things I love about living here.

On this particular afternoon, however, I wasn't thinking about crip politics; I was just happy to be spending some time bullshitting with a dear friend. I began detailing the latest developments (and sadly, non-developments) in my love life. Alana offered her usual sage advice, then chimed in with her own considerable efforts in love and lust. She was regaling me with tales of meeting her latest potential love interest, just getting to the good part, when I noticed, out of the corner of my eye, a woman standing over our table. "Umm—I just wanted to let the two of you know that I think this is really great—" she began. "I think it's so important that you are getting out in the world."

Immediately, my internal Smartass hijacked my brain: She was only an ignorant person making a stupid comment, but all I could see were Christopher Reeve and Jerry Lewis walking in, arm-in-arm, to say hello. Wanting to prevent a nasty comment from escaping my lips, I turned to Alana for help, but she wore the same "What the fuck?!" expression on her face that I felt on mine. Looking up at the woman, I recognized the misty-eyed gaze of blind crip-adoration, and my mind flashed back to other times I had been on the receiving end of similarly misguided idolatry.

Once, while riding the F-Market streetcar in San Francisco, a middle-aged guy in a business suit leaned over and commended me for my bravery: "Wow. You've got a lot of courage, kid. I don't know if I could live like that." His admiration did not translate into offering me his seat, as I stood clutching the handle above my head, struggling for balance while the streetcar shook and lurched down Market Street. Not that I would have taken it anyway. Better to risk Death by Streetcar than take the guy's pity seat.

I looked the woman in the eye and was showered with that all-too-familiar gaze once more. She didn't have to say anything; her eyes told me everything I needed to know. To her, my friend and I were brave, courageous and (goddamn I hate this word) inspirational.

We were the poor little cripples, who, through infinite inner reserves of character and saintliness, were standing up and showing the world what brave and admirable creatures we were. Dare I burst her bubble of inspiration by pointing out that we were, in actuality, bored, underpaid social services workers seizing a few precious moments to bitch about our jobs and our unfulfilled sex lives?

"I had a brother," the woman droned on. "He had Down's. We realized early on how important it was to take him out. To make sure that he got out sometimes. Right up until the end, we made sure that he got out in public." Her weird tone set my evil brain into cynical overdrive: What, exactly, did she mean by "take him out," and did it have anything to do with "the end"? No, no, no. I kicked my brain: "Drop the Tarantino script or you'll send us both to Hell."

What I wanted to say was "Gee lady, you're fucking great, but why should I care? And why do you feel the need to tell a couple of strangers how wonderful you are for treating your brother like a human being?" Instead, I only nodded, stupefied by her bizarre monologue. I turned to Alana again for help, but she was grinning at me with her "I can't believe this is happening" look.

Our admirer was still at it, yammering on about how wonderful and important it was that we were out in public view. That way, people could see us and see how "normal" we were. You'd think we had escaped from somewhere, were engaging in some noble form of social protest. Then I realized that from her perspective we were being noble and virtuous. Me, I was just trying to enjoy a cool drink and cooler company. But damn it, there we had to go and be inspirational to someone.

She finally finished her sermon about how wonderful and inspiring she found us, and went to the counter to order her drink. I turned to Alana. "That was really hard. I was this close to saying something shitty." My friend, well aware of my tendencies toward smart-assery, just grinned.

"You know," she said, "no matter how many times I get weird comments from people, it always sort of freaks me out. Were we supposed to respond? Say 'Thank you'?"

"I don't know," I said, laughing at the ridiculousness of the situation. If being a crip has taught me anything, it's taught me that a sense of humor is crucial.

"If she comes back, I want to talk to her," Alana said, eyes gleaming with wicked resolve. "I want to know why she felt the need to come over here and say that. Does she think that will make us happy, because someone thinks we're brave? Are we supposed to know that she's cool, that she 'gets it'?"

We never did get answers to any of our questions. The woman picked up her latte at the end of the counter and headed upstairs to the second floor of the café, where, I noticed, she sat down with a direct sight line to our table. She seemed to forget the newspaper she held in her hand as she gazed down at us with a mixture of awe and admiration.

* * *

Thinking about this episode, I can't help but wonder about that woman. She never came back to our table. Alana never got to play Velma to my Fred in a game of Scooby Doo detective. What did she want from us? How were we supposed to respond? Does she realize that her comments were strange at best, patronizing and offensive at worst?

We weren't doing anything out of the ordinary, just

trying to enjoy some all-too-scarce time hanging out. Yet, to this woman, we were utterly remarkable. It makes me sad that despite all the strides disabled people are making, we're still seen as admirable just for being. Even in Berkeley, some people still find our presence noteworthy. I can't speak for anyone else, but as someone who always gets remembered as "the crippled guy," I would be perfectly happy to be anonymous and unremarkable, just for once.

All my life, (nondisabled) people have been amazed, inspired, and filled with admiration at my very existence. Are any of those emotions real, or are they the polite code words for what people really feel: fear, pity, dread, and shame at the fact that they can hear themselves thinking, "Oh, God, I hope I never end up like that."

I don't need to be anyone's poster-boy. I don't want to inspire anybody, unless I actually do something great. In fact, amongst my crippled cronies, the word inspire has come to be something of an epithet. If one of my friends needs a good poke in the ribs, I can just insert a faux-heartfelt, "Yeah, and you're so inspiring to me today." Then we laugh.

The question is: Why are we laughing? Is it because that tired gag is funny, or is it because we're so goddamn sick of being special and admirable and courageous and . . . inspirational that we have to laugh to keep from thinking about how much further we all have to go?

Wings of Wax

Michael Raymond

The stumps' dull throbs sharpen and shoot up Stephen's thighs. The jolts of hot piercing pain sicken him. The fifty-two year-old double amputee sits up, pivots on the mattress, and hoists himself onto the wheelchair.

In the kitchen, Joyce glances up from her *Travel & Leisure* magazine with a cover of a muscular para-sailor soaring over the Mediterranean Sea. A long sip of coffee doesn't quite disguise her flicker of irritation with her husband's intrusion.

"You're up early."

"The medication isn't doing the trick anymore."

Joyce hides behind her magazine.

"What's on your agenda today?"

"Help you, and then run some errands."

"Good coffee."

"Same ol' same ol."

A series of piercing spasms disturbs his pleasure in the hot, bitter coffee. He spins around and wheels toward the study, bumping into the wall and gouging paint off the molding. In the study, Stephen rubs the aching stumps. He hears the garage door opening. The van's engine turns over and revs three times. As Joyce backs out, the mechanical garage door clamps down.

"Taking off? Enjoy your damn errands."

Stephen bristles with the pain. He can't work. Leaving the manuscript untouched, he negotiates into the guest bedroom. As he struggles into boxer shorts, khaki pants, and a short-sleeved black knit shirt, the rocking and straining trigger sharp stabs from the phantom left foot. Stephen swears and grits his teeth. He waits, hanging listlessly like the rolled pant cuffs below his knees. Keys, wallet, and a urinal are stuffed into a backpack. The double amputee rolls through the narrow hallway, across the living room, around the dining room table, down a small ramp, and to the back of the house.

He sets his brakes to unlock the back door. A larger ramp launches Stephen into the backyard. The gate whacks him twice in the knees before he gets through the cyclone fence.

"I'm out of here."

Dead leaves and pine needles cover the clay-and-shell driveway that slopes to the road. Stephen muscles the wheelchair through the soft clay and thick mud. At the driveway's crest, he locks the brakes to rest his aching arms.

"No sense in being a hood ornament."

Stephen hears only his labored breathing as the chair creeps to the road's edge. Glancing in both directions, he rolls into the street and hurriedly wheels up the Miller's driveway. The stumps are on fire. A steep grade stretches between Stephen and Powers Drive. He holds his breath and focuses on getting the heavy wheelchair moving over the cracked sidewalk. He leans forward and pulls, and pulls, and pulls. Shoulder and arm pain slows him as he strains up the hill.

Drenched in sweat, Stephen stops at Powers Drive. His chest heaves as he studies the traffic. The chair rolls down into the gutter. Stephen seizes the first opening between speeding cars. Coasting to the middle, he waits on the middle double line. Vehicles whiz by. His head swivels left and right. A white Tempo comes up fast on the inside lane. An Explorer and a plumber's truck sweep by. Stephen grunts and pushes down on the hard rubber wheels. The chair rolls toward a driveway as a train of cars undulates up and down the busy road.

Turning west, Stephen wrestles the wheelchair up and down the hills and valleys on Powers. Patches of sand bog down the chair. A bicyclist nearly clips him. Cars honk. Stephen's body aches and melts with the rising temperature and the work. The sidewalk ends at the mall. Traffic sits at the parking lot's entrance. Stephen sweats and waits. Pain sears his arms and stumps. Five, ten, fifteen minutes pass. The entrance remains choked. After ten more minutes, a woman in a maroon Escort stops, honks, and motions him in. Stephen waves before scuttling into the mall's parking lot.

A familiar white van sits in a designated disabled parking spot at the mall entrance.

"That's curious. I wonder."

Banging through the two sets of doors, Stephen wheels smoothly past Swan Dry Cleaners and Champion Rent-to-Own. Shoppers smile at him outside the specialty clothing stores, Stepp Office Supply, and Walgreen's. Their kids stare.

The wheelchair speeds to the end of one concourse, past a Subway franchise and The Muse Bookstore, to Apollo's Pub. As Stephen reaches out, a Consolidated Power & Light employee holds open the pub's door without looking at the legless pants.

"Thanks."

Scattered tables with dirty dishes cluster in the middle. A few patrons occupy clean tables. Dark booths line the pub's walls.

"I'll be damned."

Joyce sits in the back booth with *Travel & Leisure*, a glass, and a half-full bottle of wine.

"You alone?"

Joyce's head snaps up. She pauses.

"Buy you a drink, stranger? Looks like you could use one."

"Sure."

As Joyce goes for another glass, Stephen hoists himself into the booth. He folds up the wheelchair and pushes it behind the booth.

"Come here often, mister?"

"I don't get out much."

She fills his glass.

"Here's to new places."

"To Byzantium." They drink.

"You look beat, Mr. Hicks. You just break out of prison?"

"Something like that. A paltry thing. A sail in a gale."

"On the run?"

"So to speak. What's your story?"

Joyce drains her wine.

"I'm waiting, wondering. Hiding out."

"From?"

"A trashy lot."

"It's a man, isn't it?"

"Maybe. It's been a terrible fall, and a worse spring."

"Not putting his best foot forward?"

"Stephen, that's awful!"

"Tell him to shake a leg."

"That's terrible. You're terrible."

"This guy clearly hasn't got a leg to stand on."

"Stop!"

Stephen pours the last of the wine.

"Joyce, it's been rough. I feel trapped. I know I said I'd be back, that everything would be better. I feel like I'm drowning. I can't seem to re-invent myself. I'm sorry."

"I know. It's like our life's over. I take you to the office, you work, I drag you home. You don't go out, we don't do anything. You . . ."

"I'm sorry."

"I'd give anything for you to have your legs back, but I feel we're both trapped."

"I know." Stephen leans forward, reaching to rub his legs.

"Hey, who gave you a ride? How'd you get here?"

"No one. I rolled myself."

"That's a long way."

"Long and hot. I may never lift my arms again."

"And dangerous. How'd you get across Powers?"

"My chair has wings. We were spectacular. A nearly flawless flight. From now on, the chair and I are inseparable."

"A mighty duo."

"Indeed. Sound the trumpets. We conquered—let's see, a hill and a vale, a perilous crossing of the Rubicon, and made a desperate flight to freedom."

"A girl should be proud to drink with two such desperados."

"Heroes. We didn't blink. We didn't cringe."

"Ah, now I see those massive steel arms and the shoulders of a god."

"At the very least."

"How can the world turn away? They should celebrate your heroic deeds. Cheer your amazing feat . . ."

"Feat? Feet. Get it?" Stephen lifts his stumps into view and waggles them.

"Stop, that's not funny. None of this is funny."

"What is then?"

"I don't know, but it isn't funny. Are you finished with your wine? Let's get out of here. I'll take you home."

Stephen drags himself down the bench. He reaches back for his wheelchair. It bangs against the booth. He leans over precariously, unfolds the chair, places it parallel to the booth, and locks the brakes.

"You want some help?"

"No. No, thank you."

Stephen places his left hand on the far wheel and his right hand on the bench. In one slow, careful motion, he lifts his half body up and swings the stumps over the front of the wheelchair. He eases his body down and drags it over the wheel into the seat. His cuffed pants catch on the chair's protruding knob. He frees himself and settles into the wheelchair.

Joyce is gone. He eases himself past abandoned chairs, around crowded tables, and through milling customers. The stumps throb.

"Tower, this is Flight 063 . . ."

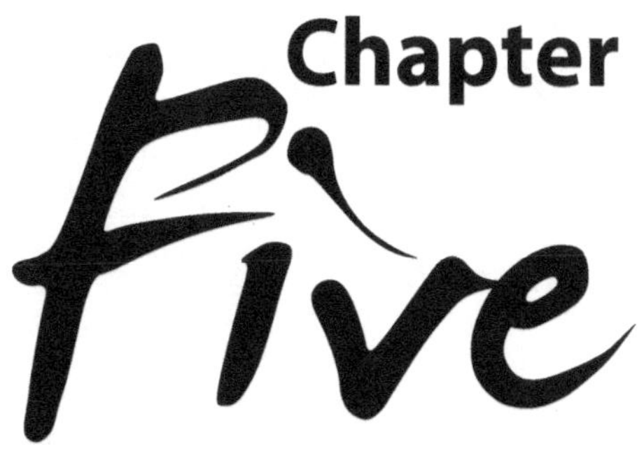

Integration, Distraction, and Recreation

In the beginning, illness and disability often take center stage. They demand all of our energy and redefine our life goals. At some point, we find a way to transition back to our everyday activities—even when dealing with a serious illness. We learn to integrate our health issues so they become a backdrop to the richness of our lives.

I Am Not My Body

Glenn Reitz

I am not my body
I am not weak,
weak with fatigue,
weak with atrophy,
weak with limbs that give out well before the job is done.

I am not my body
I am not dying,
decaying, degenerating, debilitating, disease-ridden,
dissolving, disappearing . . .

slowly, like blood stains on the sidewalk, bleaching
under footsteps and the daily sun—
until one day you realize that they're gone
and can't remember who bled, who died.
All you do remember
is that the crime scene jammed traffic for blocks,
the sudden stop/ start of the bus
spilling coffee on your shirt and
making you late for work.
You remember that.
Curious, though, the coffee stain is still there no matter what you do—
just keep your jacket closed so no one sees.

I am not my body
slipping slowly into shadows
Losing brightness and luminosity
Sinking in obscurity and the susurrus of memory.

I am not my body
slowly wearing out like an eraser on the pencil of a writer
leaving bits and pieces of myself behind, evidence of mistakes and
redirected thought,
wearing slowly to a useless nub.

> If I would write less perhaps I would last longer,
> maintain my shape,
> my form,
> my body
> but the writing serves a purpose, if only to make the eraser useful.
> And the writing I can't stop.

I am not my body
I'm a shining, luminous creature,
casting shadows of my own illuminescence
burning into minds and onto paper
growing stronger every day.
New appetites feed cravings—new expressions—wings of thought,
imparting flight like that of hummingbirds—no,

not stupid hummingbirds but honeybees.
Swarming out from hidden places, taking
sustenance and energy
from everywhere they stop to feed,
yet leaving pollen, fertile and productive,
bits and pieces left behind. They, too, serve a
purpose.
But even bees are gone at sunset, fly to shadows
'fore the night arrives

So maybe then I'm not a bee, or hummingbird.
But I am damned sure not my body

Recycling Soles

Jennifer Kern

They were not the greatest hiking boots, but I bought them with my own money, and they did the job. All emerging feminists in the eighties needed army surplus wool pants and hiking boots. I did, anyway. Even with the hem out, the pants barely brushed the laces, though the boots boldly filled the gap. Size nine looked bigger in beige, and wider somehow. They were stiff at first and weighed enough to exaggerate my confidence.

In the autumn woods behind our house, affectionately known as "The Outhouse," Dan and I had our final marathon breakup session. I paced and stood digging my booted feet into the earth while declaring my independence: Who needs feminist rhetoric when she's got hiking boots with black laces? I can stand on my own two feet, thank you.

As I moved through The Outhouse in the days that followed, the mud that clogged the waffle tread littered the floors of the kitchen, the bathroom, and the hallway. I made a mess breaking in the stiff leather while toughening my aching feet and wounded heart. Each dirt dropping, a memory turd of our dissolution in the woods.

During that winter break in Vermont, those bulky boots kept me ten-toed and warm enough—even without waterproofing. Permitting two pair of bulky wool socks, they protected my feet from the towering snowdrifts that buried windowsills and woodpiles.

As I trudged through the snow, I thought: With these boots, can fit in here. I am a survivor. I can do the job.

In the aftermath of that January ice storm, my boots and I crunched two miles up the hill from the bus station to The Outhouse. Burdened under the weight of my overstuffed backpack, I sweated as I hiked, breathing in the sun-induced thaw, leaving indomitable snowwoman tracks behind me. The trees sagged with icicle branches that glistened and creaked like aging limbs.

On that day, the sun was blinding in its brilliance, the snow drifts a mere prop for its reflection. Below the crunchy shell, the soggy snow encrusted my laces and settled in my cuffs. Not a soul was in sight in that winter wonder world. Those boots did a great job that day—my last winter hike before wheels replaced those boots of mine. It's imprinted on my brain like skid marks left on a heart.

I did not cry when I gave my boots to my sister Ann that summer after the accident. They were not the greatest hiking boots. I would miss my running shoes more. Most of all, I'd miss making snow angels.

They did the job for me, those old boots, and now they are Ann's. I hope she waterproofed them.

Elvis Lives

Maggie Jochild

In December of 2001, two dear friends who "get it" rescued me from spending Christmas absolutely alone by sending me a plane ticket to visit them in Boston. All I had to do was get myself physically there and back. But that was the part that made me anxious. This would be the first time I had flown since my knee replacement surgery. I can't stand for very long, can walk only short distances, need to change positions often, run a high risk of blood clots in my legs, don't fit in most airline seats, get asthma in pressurized cabins . . . I was, well, anxious.

But if you think I was anxious—this was just a few months after 9/11. I would be flying into cold, grey, paranoid Logan Airport, the airport that launched United flight 175 and American flight 11. To add to their burden, the day I traveled was the day a lunatic tried to set off explosives in his tennis shoes and *that* flight was emergency landed at Logan.

Passengers were being separated from their loved ones right away. After that point, I would be in a wheelchair and, like Blanche Dubois, relying on the kindness of strangers—strangers wearing dark blue American Airlines blazers and stony faces. I kept telling everybody, at every step of the way, that I needed an extra-wide wheelchair. Apparently, Logan couldn't find such a thing, so I was crammed into what I think of as the California surfer girl model. But then, my luck turned. A tall young man with a full beard stepped forward from the cluster of blue blazers to be my official escort: Enter Ahmed.

Ahmed was from Saudi Arabia, from a city that had been home to two of the hijackers. His looks, his accent, his absolute being made all the passengers in the airport freeze up around him. He was fucking sick of it. And here I was, a huge crippled dyke. If we were dumped out of a car together into the town square of an average small white burg, I don't know which one of us would get stoned to death first. We bonded instantly.

Turns out, in his off hours Ahmed was an Elvis impersonator. I don't know how he got around the obstacle of his beard, but in terms of dialogue, he really had it down. My little brother Bill was also an Elvis impersonator, so Ahmed found in me the perfect foil. I'd feed him a line like "Melli Kalikimakki" and he'd start singing "I'll have a buh-looo Crismuss without yew." I'd ask him which part of Boston he lives in, he'd break into "Since mah baybee left me / Ah found a new place to dwell . . ."

Ahmed as Elvis was charming, and clearly disconcerting to his fellow American Airlines employees. He didn't seem to give a rat's ass. He kept trying to find ways for me to get through the long lines and bottlenecks faster. At checkpoints, even though the wheelchair I was in was clearly their property, I had to get up and walk while they removed this chair and replaced it with another—also their property. Looking around at all these humorless guys in camouflage carrying assault rifles, I had to wonder, what is it that I could pull off in a wheelchair that would be as deadly as those automatic weapons. I mean, I'm not a crip McGyver.

They also seemed to be stopping people randomly and asking them to remove their shoes for inspection. We didn't know about the sneaker bomber yet, so this struck Ahmed and me as especially hilarious. I can get my shoes off by myself, but not back on without certain kinds of help. I decided if they picked me, Ahmed could use the occasion of kneeling before me to do the proposal scene from *Viva Las Vegas.*

My friend Danny, who is wheelchair-bound and Latino, also had to fly somewhere this same holiday season. He told me later that when he was selected out for a shoe search, he was honored that he could still be perceived as a possible terrorist, even though he was an overt cripple. Then he added that what probably pushed him over the edge from pity into menace was the spic factor.

When I went through the metal detector, I told the guys on this end of it that my left knee is titanium and it absolutely would set off the alarm. Even so, when I emerged on the other side, the quality of what registered on their security monitor brought every blue blazer in the vicinity to stand around me. Ahmed waved at me over the shoulder of one official. I emptied all my pockets, but I was still setting off red rockets of alarms. But Logan was running short on the little wands they use to wave over people's bodies, so I had to be patted down by a security expert. They sent for the one woman apparently allowed to do this kind of work.

Now, here's the thing. I am a lesbian Chandler Bing; I make jokes when I am nervous. I was nervous then.

They were keeping Ahmed and the second wheelchair a few feet away, giving me a folding chair to sit on until the pat-down artist arrived. And when they parted the blue blazers to let her through, she was—of course—skinny, white, extremely straight, with impeccable makeup and hair. Except when I'm in all-lesbian groups, I have never in my life been wearing the right clothes around other women. She looked as dismayed at the sight of me as I was at the sight of her.

So, I had some tension to let off. I managed to keep it together until she reached a certain region that my mother referred to as munchkin land, as in, "Did you wash good in munchkin land?" Which made watching *The Wizard of Oz* a truly bizarre experience as a child . . . but I digress. When her pale, well-manicured hands began searching munchkin land for box cutters or plastic explosives, I could not help myself. I said, with complete Tupelo charm: "Thank yew, thank yew verra much."

Replacement Players

Floyd Skloot

I thought, *why not?* I wasn't doing anything else at the time. It was only a four hour drive up to Seattle, where the Mariners were holding their tryout camp at the Kingdome, and we'd just put new tires on the car.

Didn't look like the players and owners would settle the strike in time for spring training, so the teams were all holding winter tryout camps. Sure, I was in my late forties, but they were talking about bringing back players older than that. I'd seen pictures in the paper of guys who looked as though they'd gained more weight since retiring than I weighed altogether, guys who had a lot more gray hair than I do under the 1911 New York Yankees cap my wife Meredith got me for Valentine's Day. Hell, I've had gray hair since I was twenty nine, especially in my beard. I kept walking around the house singing that old Crosby, Stills and Nash song, *what have I got to lose?*

For the past six years, I'd been disabled by a rare neurological disorder, one of those diseases that's named after the physician who discovered it but died before he could figure out how to cure the thing. Still, it was something that could be controlled most of the time. As long as I didn't get too fatigued, and didn't try to do too much at any one time or for too long, and provided that I followed a few simple management procedures, most of the symptoms could be held in check. Sometimes my world listed a bit to the left, but I'd learned how to compensate for that. In the batter's box, hitting curve balls could be tricky, because they'd probably make me dizzy, but lots of guys can't hit curve balls. Out at second base, I might have trouble going back under a pop fly, especially if I put my arms out to the side while looking up at the ball the way I was trained to do, because then I'd simply fall down. Same thing if I had my feet together and closed my eyes, but once I got past the national anthem I couldn't imagine a time I'd do that during the game. There could also be some difficulty with the coach's signals, since my short-term memory is pretty erratic these days, or concentrating if the fans made too much noise. But I figured I could face those problems when I got to them. Besides, there probably wouldn't be too many fans anyway.

Look, I'll be honest, I could use the money. What I get from Social Security and from my former employer makes it so we eat a lot of tuna-helper after about the twenty-third of the month. Plus, I used to play some ball, back before I got sick. Actually, back before I graduated from college, but the big league scouts were always around and I thought I had a shot until that one game where I struck out five times. Still. Meredith and I always went up to watch the Mariners play several times a season and I have to tell you I could play as well as some of those jokers. Meredith says so too and she hasn't even seen me play. But she has seen me at the batting ranges, where I can still spray line drives from both sides of the plate. I never lost the touch, even in the cages with the 80 mph machines. The way I figure it, there won't be too many guys throwing faster than that among the replacement players.

But it's not just the money, of course. Playing big-league ball is something I always dreamed of doing, ever since I was a kid in Brooklyn, New York, going to Ebbets Field to watch the Dodgers. I have very clear memories of being there in 1957, sitting just to the first base side of home plate, watching the Dodgers finish out their Brooklyn lives. Across the left field wall there were all those signs—The Brass Rail, Schaefer Beer, Luckies, Buy Tydol—and then Gino Cimoli or Sandy Amoros beside the 351 ft. sign against left handed batters. Yeah, I would be happy with just one game, one time at bat, one grounder cleanly fielded.

When we pulled into the Kingdome parking lot that morning, I thought, *well I guess I'm not the only one.* Meredith just laughed once, that wonderful guffaw of hers, then got hold of herself and wove her way through the crowded lot to the handicapped parking area right next to the entrance. She seemed as happy as I was.

"Maybe you'd better leave your cane in the car," she said.

This was something I'd already thought of myself. I mean, give me some credit. I zipped open my bag and checked everything one more time: mitt, shoes, batting gloves, new shoes, lucky tee shirt, the small crystal Meredith gave me for luck. I took a couple of my noon hour pills a little early, so no one would have to see me doing it inside, and we were ready to go. She leaned over to give me a kiss, then tugged down her Mariners cap, slipped on her Joe Carter mitt so she could catch foul balls, threw her sweater over her shoulders, and we got out. At the gate, she took out her camera and got a good shot of me heading down the ramp toward the clubhouse.

"Break a leg, Shooter," she shouted after me. Meredith used to be an actress and she doesn't know much about baseball, but that didn't stop her from giving me her full support. Or using the wrong nickname. On the ride up to Seattle, I'd confessed that in school my teammates called me Scooter.

Getting to the clubhouse was like passing through customs at the airport in Damascus. Once they were sure I didn't have any contraband in my bag, and once I'd spent a half hour filling out all their forms—no, I wouldn't sue the Mariners if I died as a result of the tryout—and trying not to exaggerate my baseball accomplishments, I was given number 49 to pin on my shirt and waved through to the inner sanctum. I don't think anyone saw me bump into the door jamb as I walked in.

The only thing that surprised me about the locker room was how small it seemed. I thought modern players had all these contractual agreements giving them a quarter mile of airspace between each other or something. Hot tubs and massage tables and a spate of nautilus machines. I thought there would be director's chairs or padded recliners by every locker.

I also thought there would be a more even distribution among the guys who were trying out. But most of them, a good eighty percent or more, were half my age, a few of them polite enough not to stare and then turn back to their lockers gagging down their laughter. But only a few. There seemed to be a grandfather's corner over by the coach's office, where I saw three guys who probably could remember Timothy Leary or knew Frankie Lymon and the Teenagers weren't a neighborhood gang. They were carefully pulling on their stirrup socks and lacing their shoes, none of which were as clean as mine.

"Hey, how you doing?" I said, trying to sound crusty. Also trying to keep my vocabulary simple enough so I wouldn't end up saying the wrong word. Earlier in the day, I'd generously informed Meredith that we were in the *excerpts* of Seattle instead of the *outskirts*.

One of the younger older guys knocked his bag off a stool and shoved the rickety three-legger over toward me. Another guy opened a locker next to the one he was using and took out his equipment so I could use the locker. The third member of the group looked familiar enough that I wondered if he was a retired player, somebody whose face I'd seen in *The Sporting News* a few years back.

"No," he said, before I asked. "I just look like the fella. Odell Jones. He played for six different teams in nine years and had the absolute worst season of his illustrious career right here in Seattle. The General Manager called me 'Odell' when he came by a few minutes ago and said he was glad to see me back. I just shook his hand and nodded—far be it from me to correct the man. Maybe I'll make the team if I keep my mouth shut around the coaching staff. Later they'll be too embarrassed to drop me."

"What did I miss so far?" I asked.

"Nothing," the guy who was not Odell Jones said. "No one said a thing to us all morning. Except the little old clubhouse guy keeps telling us not to throw anything on the floor and if we have the runs we should clean the throne ourselves. That notice over by the water cooler says tryouts begin at eleven."

I guessed I should be able to get my shoes tied in the next half hour, especially if I didn't try to talk at the same time, so I nodded and turned toward my locker. A few of the younger men were filing out and heading toward a passage that must have led onto the field. Within three minutes, the place was deserted except for the three of us geezers.

The one sitting next to me started talking as though we'd been having a conversation all morning. "So I told her you can come or you can stay, makes no difference to me, but I'm going to Seattle. You know what she does?" He looked at me, his socks dangling from both hands as though he wasn't sure whether to put them on or use them to strangle me.

I shook my head and started searching diligently for my Yankees cap.

"Only closes down the bank account, packs up and drives to her mother in Sacramento, that's all. I had to take the damn train up here and borrow a hundred bucks from my brother. How am I supposed to play major league quality ball when she does this to me? I don't make the team now, I know whose fault it is."

"Shoot," not-Odell Jones said. "My old lady doesn't know where I'm at. Probably thinks I took off for some meeting and forgot to leave her a note. She's cool."

"What do you do?" I asked, mostly as an excuse to turn away from my neighbor, who was still staring at me, maybe wondering if I had given his wife the idea about Sacramento.

"Software. I write those manuals tell you how to use a

program. And play in the softball leagues around town. I hit 91 homers last summer."

"Was relaxed, I could hit me a few taters," my neighbor mumbled. "I could probably hit one clear out of this place. Say, any you guys got something help a person relax?"

Finally the oldest of us, the one who hadn't said anything yet, slammed his locker shut and turned to the rest of us. He had on an old Seattle Pilots hat and a purple University of Washington sweat suit, and his face was all grim lines and odd shadows, like a charcoal sketch of a cubist portrait. His high voice was a shock coming out of such a long, cowboy body.

"You know what this is?" He waited, a professor giving us adult ed students plenty of time to frame our answers, then sadly nodded as though he knew all along how dumb we really were. "Only the most important day of my life, that's all. I am not here to dink around, get cut and go back to Yakima so I can tell my drinking buddies about my grand adventure. This is no adolescent fantasy for me, so I don't want to hear any more talk about your fastballs and your home runs. I've had enough." He stalked out of the locker room, pounding a ball into his mitt, and we could still hear him talking as he disappeared from view.

Not-Odell Jones looked at my neighbor, who was tying his shoes, and then at me. He shrugged. "I hope they got a doctor on call."

I waited till the other two oldsters had left, saying I needed a couple minutes in private, and went over to the full length mirror by the showers. Hate to say this, but I really looked all right, if a little tired around the eyes.

You'd never know I was brain-damaged, especially if I wasn't trying to copy your movements or follow complicated directions. Last month, to get me in shape for this, Meredith bought an exercise video and we popped it into the VCR. Here were these supple young kids hopping around behind a woman who looked a lot like not-Odell Jones, and she was hollering out directions, saying *now turn left* while turning to my right, saying *right arm to left ankle* like we're playing 'Simon Says' but then dropping the arm that was on my left, till I just had to sit down on the couch and watch Meredith rock n' roll.

Anyway, I looked all right, so I picked up a bat that was leaning against the first locker by the door. I took my usual lefty batting stance and glared at an imaginary pitcher, then shifted my weight and took a smooth inside-out cut, the bat ending up in my right hand pointing toward the bathroom, a perfect swing. I was ready.

At the mouth of the stairway leading into the dugout, I practiced what my occupational therapist had taught me long ago. I stopped to get my bearings, noticing the layout before me, the obstacles in my path, and studied the steps up onto the field. *Four short steps,* I told myself. That way I would have a better chance of not falling on my face.

When I trotted out to the field, I could clearly hear Meredith screaming for me from behind the dugout. She was using one of those high-pitched calls like middle eastern women give out, her tongue flapping wildly against the roof of her mouth to make a little trilling sound. Maybe I'd stumbled into a belly dancing contest instead of a baseball tryout. I knew she was snapping pictures too. If I wasn't being so cool, I would have trotted over and given her a kiss of thanks for steady support.

As soon as I crossed into the outfield, not-Odell Jones tossed a ball to me. I caught it and threw it back before realizing that I was thinking about something else, about how hard the astroturf felt and how strangely sound moved down there on the playing field. Damn, I was lucky the ball didn't hit me in the face.

"Feeling all right?" I yelled to him. But he wouldn't answer. I'd forgotten that he didn't want to speak in front of the coaches. "Sorry."

They broke us into two groups of about forty each, half moving toward the left field foul line and half toward right. These were the sprints. We had to run past these old guys with stopwatches, scouts or personnel staff or auditors, I don't know who they were.

I hadn't thought about having to race. Let me hit, fellas. Let me field some grounders. I used to be fast. I used to have all my hair, too, but those were qualities that I was losing before I got sick. Hey, forty yards isn't that far, right?

When the whistle blew, I got a good start and simply refused to let myself look anywhere but at the ground right in front of me. Good thing Meredith and I had jogged together to the mailbox and back all month, an easy quarter mile, because my leg muscles were in fairly decent shape now and I didn't pull anything. Amazing: I got past the scouts in just under six seconds. Everybody who came in over six seconds had to run it again and after three tries was dismissed from the tryout. I immediately went to the center field wall and sat with my back against it, watching the action. Not-Odell Jones made it on his second try, as did the guy from Yakima. I saw my neighbor walking toward the dugout with his mitt on his head like a cap and was doubly thrilled not to be going to the locker room.

After the speed test, there were about fifty of us left. We had to throw to each other, one group standing at the outfield wall, the other standing just beyond the infield dirt. Twenty minutes later there were about forty left.

I was getting very tired and hoped they'd let me hit while I could still stand. They split us into three groups this time, sending ten toward home plate for their turns at bat and splitting the rest into pitchers, who went to the bullpen with a coach, and fielders who had to catch whatever came their way. Fortunately, I was among the ten. The fielders had to concentrate not only on what we hit, but also on balls being hit to them by coaches. I didn't want to think about having to go out there after my turn at bat.

Suddenly I heard Meredith cheering for me again. She'd moved from behind the dugout to behind home plate. I hadn't heard a thing for the last half hour.

The guy from Yakima took his place in the batter's box. He looked good up there, the bat waggling high above his head, his knees slightly flexed. I was impressed, but the batting practice pitcher wasn't—the first pitch was very close to his head and sent him reeling backwards out of the box.

I could just imagine him saying "I've had enough." He dug in exactly where he'd been standing before and started waggling the bat again. The next pitch, a low fastball, he golfed into deep left field, a major league shot. He hit the next one directly back at the pitcher, who was protected by a screen but nevertheless ducked automatically, which set loose a round of friendly jeering from the coaches. Yakima was impressive; he drilled the next three pitches, one each to left, center, and right. On his last swing, he gave it everything he had, the angriest and most ferocious cut I ever hope to see. The ball went straight up and seemed to get lost in the gray paint of the dome before reappearing as it came down behind third base. He stormed out of the box toward the outfield, cursing himself for overswinging, and made a wide loop around the coaches. I never saw him again.

When it was my turn to hit, I found myself both relaxed and fully focused. Better get through it before things start swirling on me. The pitcher was lefthanded, so I went over to hit right-handed, which was always my better side anyway. Things were falling into place. The first pitch went by so fast I didn't have time to notice anything except the hiss the ball made in the instant before it popped into the catcher's mitt. I stepped out to regain my composure, squeezed the bat between my hands, adjusted my batting gloves, and stepped back in. The next pitch was a hard curve, which I could see fairly well but didn't even think about swinging at. As the ball broke downwards and out of the strike zone, I followed the flight with my eyes, almost staggering across the plate after it. If this was *The Gong Show*, I thought, I was about to get gonged. What was with this pitcher? Was he still mad at my friend from Yakima and taking it out on me?

His next pitch was a fastball, but slightly slower than the first one and I swung at it, fouling the pitch straight back. It looped directly toward the area where Meredith had been standing. I spun around to watch it, losing my balance and teetering toward third base, but could just see her reach up with her gloved hand and catch the ball before I hit the ground. Oh man, we got a souvenir, bless her sweet soul.

"Nice swing, 49," someone yelled from behind me. "Now straighten it out."

I dusted myself off and got ready to step back in. Suddenly I realized that, whatever else happened today, it didn't really matter. I was exhausted and dizzy, but I had done it. With Meredith's help, I'd come up to Seattle when it didn't seem like I'd ever be able to travel again. I'd made it most of the way through the tryouts, had gotten to hit and made contact with a good fastball. We had pictures and a ball to take home with us, but of course that wasn't really the point. The point was what was now inside my head, along with the bizarre image now forming of the pitching mound as it drifted toward third base. Indeed, the entire field was beginning to rearrange itself in my vision, as fields do when I am tired, and I knew it was time to call it quits.

I looked out toward the center field stands, where Meredith and I preferred sitting so we could catch home runs during Mariners games, though we'd never actually managed to snag one. Then I took a deep breath and, using the bat as a cane, walked over to the stands behind home plate. By the time I got there, Meredith had come down toward the field and was waiting for me, arms wide, tears in her eyes, her face open in an enormous smile.

I waved the next batter into the box, then made my way slowly into the locker room to shower and change. As I was drying myself, not-Odell Jones came in and slumped on the stool in front of his locker.

"Cat's out of the bag," he said. "Even with my mouth shut, they figured out I wasn't Odell Jones as soon as they saw I threw lefty."

"That's too bad."

"I told them I hit 91 homers last summer. But it was too late, man."

"Did you get to bat?"

"Yeah, but I left my stroke home. Hit nothing but air."

I took his phone number and promised to call sometime. His real name was Reese Morgan and he lived less than an hour from us. I thought Meredith would like him. She was waiting for me at the main gate, popping the ball I'd hit into her glove and singing her favorite song, "Try a Little Tenderness." She didn't hear me coming because of the echo her voice made in the concrete hallway. I snatched the ball out of the air, backed up a step, bent at the knees and joined her in song: "You got to, you got to, you got to . . ."

from
Home Grown

Riua Akinshegun

This is an excerpt from a collection of letters from Georgetown, Guyana to Home Grown. Home Grown is anyone who comes from where I was born or anyone who can understand my journey.

Dear Home Grown,

Oh, yes, I did get to the Stabroek Market. It is full of fruits and vegetables, strangely beautiful—colors and smells that would make an artist's palette envious. The bustling of the people, the bartering, just pulls you right in. La! La!

But that is not what's on my mind right now—my wheelchair is down again.

I had started my search for musicians to accompany me in a reading. Everyone told me I wouldn't be able to find a blues guitarist, but there was a guitarist who could play the blues. I was pointed to the Sidewalk Cafe, the only jazz club in Guyana.

It was Thursday night. The house band was jamming—playing to a packed crowd of mostly "been to" (Guyanese who have been abroad) and ex-patriots. The musicians' demeanor, their dress, their slow walk across the stage, and their preoccupation with the musicians' muse—tit tit tit tap taps on half-filled beer bottles and tabletops—was universal.

The pianist, a short stout man with stubby fingers you wouldn't think could dance across a keyboard, had a twinkle in his mahogany eyes and an international following. He had moments of genius that transported us past the dominant sounds of the evening: soft jazz. The horn player that night was a renegade from the States, a Home Grown African, who came to Guyana retreating from the aftermath of the sixties. He had the appearance of a willow, lean and blowing. His trumpet solos were reaches of Miles Davis. He put my big toe back in Leimert Park, where Home Grown jazz musicians go to jam after gigging in Los Angeles's finest alleyways. The guitarist, Herbie Marshall, would die to sit in a jam session like that in our yard. He drools when he speaks of our Home Grown musicians. After the intermission, he glided onto the stage and worked in a few blues chords on his guitar for me to sample. Herbie will do just fine behind my reading, just fine, even though he rocks like a rock-and-roller. Home Grown, I even found a lead on a master drummer for *She Is Me,* my piece on how the disabled are treated in Africa.

This spot, the Sidewalk Café, could conceivably become a watering hole for me. It's eclectic, friendly, and accessible . . . It was a great night! So great that my friends and I continued on to a disco to hear a reggae band.

Home Grown, we got to the club, right? My host, Vic, who was a little bit tipsy, bounced out of the car—rhythms of jazz still playing in his ears—and headed for the trunk of his car to retrieve my chair. There was a tropical chill in the night air, yet all the windows were rolled down—we were hot to trot.

Suddenly, Vic popped back at my window like a robber, moist curl dewdrops of desperation were clinging to his mustache. He was panting as if he had just run a 100-yard dash. "Riua, your-wheelchair-is-not-there." We laughed, thinking it was the liquor dripping.

Diane sucked the wind through her teeth and teased, "Ssssssss, don't bother. I'll get it meself. Dem men dem can't do noth'in for dem self. Dem men should stay home with dem mamas." Her big-boned body leaped out of the back seat like a feather blowing in the air of a backhand dismissal. She continued, "We women has to do every . . ." Within an instant she returned with eyes expanded saucer-like. "There's no chair!"

I reached into everyone's eyes, soliciting denials: "What do you mean no chair, what?"

Diane's hands flopped with each word as if it would help me hold on to the meaning. "Gawd! Aw Gawd! There's no chair! It's not in the trunk. Oh, Gawd."

"What?!"

"It must have fallen out along the way now!"

"And we didn't hear it?!" I whimpered.

I knew Vic's car trunk wasn't quite empty; he had to maneuver things around to make room. The small wheels hung out over the bumper. The hood bounced up and down as we raced to the club, talking above the rattles. Still . . .

Can you perceive the fright I carried as we retraced our path? Before, I hadn't noticed the darkness of night, or the numerous potholes. We moved gingerly down the streets as if we were leading a procession to a wake. I felt as if I were the person they were going to bury.

I was quietly frantic. My inner conversation went:

"How will the other cars avoid my wheelchair in this dim light?" *Bump 13.* "If we can't find it, how will I go to the bathroom? What—" *bump 27* "—am I going to do? What if someone has found it and taken it home and turned it into a fruit cart? Or what if someone has run over it and killed themselves or worse, damaged my chair? What—" *bump 31* "—will I do?" Moving on three wheels was a piece of cake. Did I complain too much? Guyana without a wheelchair?

I went into a meditative rock and watched. Diane and Vic rocked in sympathy too; even the car rocked as we inched farther down the streets. Then, just before my sad face was about to break, we spotted it lying on its side. My chariot's scruffy metal grabbed hold of the stars; their union alerted Vic. We released a collective sigh—"Whew!"—becoming hilariously ecstatic, full of chatter.

I gave thanks: "I-thank-you!!!!"

Vic turned the car around. The joy of the night was back on track. We stepped into the club lit up, matching the Christmas lights strung lavishly across the outdoor patio, laughing and talking loudly.

Luckily, I was in my wheelchair because I was laughing so hard that I would've fallen down if I'd been walking.

Our mood was contagious and soon the sluggish place awakened. The band started playing an upbeat tune, a mixture of reggae and soca. It made us wanna get up on our feet. We danced, ate, drank a little too much, and shared a silly conversation that always led back to the wheelchair and my life—ha, ha, ha—without it.

A few hours later we decided to call it a night and climbed into the car for our return home. We bounced along Georgetown's cavity streets with our ears wide open. The wheelchair tumbled out again. No problem. We howled and retrieved it.

They dropped me off at my apartment—*Daylight come and me wanna go home.* I was too stimulated to sleep, so I grabbed my book and glasses to quiet my energy down. The cover was turned back on my bed. Home Grown, I was dancing over to the dresser to switch the fan on to grab a little air—*Come mister tally man, tally me banana* . . . In the middle of a finger pop—"Pop!"—my large right wheel flew across the room off beat. I was thrown to the floor, scraping my right side, bumping my head against the table, sending my bed lamp crashing to the floor. The room turned dark. For about five minutes, Home Grown, I gave up and just lay there on my wheel, massaging my temples, reassuring my heart. It was a struggle to pick up the tune—*DAY . . . D SA DAY, DE SA DE A . . . A O*—but I managed. Soreness shoved aside, I examined my chair—discovered half of my spokes torn apart and my release button damaged.

My ancestor's wings lifted me up onto my bed and I've been sitting ever since. Unstrung.

Running Shoes

Michael Wille

It has been two weeks since I've laced my shoes up, and over a month since I've had the slightest inkling of hitting the trail. Normally, only the weather can break my motivation, but even then, after enough self-coaxing, I'm out enjoying solitude in the mud and rain. I look over into my closet in disgust at the pair of filthy, tattered, mud-covered Saucony running shoes. I wonder how they ever could have brought me so much enjoyment and yet have left me with so much pain.

Two months ago, I remember coming home with the bright blue shoebox and reading the catchy slogan on the cover: "Saucony, true to the sport." "Yeah, that's me," I thought. "I am a running fool." There wasn't anything else I could think of at the time. At work, I would fade off and daydream of running on my favorite trails. When surrounded by people in a social situation, I would tell stories of races past or those soon to come. Any other time, I was actually out there putting some more miles in. I was living, breathing, eating, and sleeping the sport of running and enjoying every minute of it.

After all, I had the biggest race of my life coming up with a self-organized fund-raiser to boot. I would soon be running the Marathon des Sables, the toughest footrace on earth: seven glorious days and six lavish nights across the desert of Morocco, completely self-contained. It was an adventure run that was right up my alley, and nothing was going to stop me from success—at least not this time around.

A few days prior to my departure, I was in the studio interviewing with Peter Finch, one of the most popular voices in Bay Area radio. He said, "This web site here states that you'll suffer numerous blisters on your feet, 120 degree temperatures, and almost starve to death with the small amounts of dried food you have to carry. Tell me, Michael, why would someone want to partake in an event like this?"

My response: "Well Peter, I don't know why anyone else would want to go through all that suffering, but the reason I'm going over there is to raise money for the CCFA's kids' camp." And that's when I got to tell my story. I explained the sport of ultra-running—any race longer than a marathon—and talked about all my past races. I told the listeners how, a year ago, I was hospitalized the day before I was to step on a plane to do this very race. I talked about Crohn's and Colitis diseases, and how they affect millions of Americans, including myself, and told people about the Crohn's and Colitis Foundation of America (CCFA). I also hit them up for donations to fund the kids' camp.

I ended the interview with a bold and presumptuous statement I had used with people so many times before. I compared the suffering involved in a week of running across the Moroccan desert with a single minute spent on a hospital bed. Even though I hadn't been to Morocco, I knew from my ultra-running experience that when things started to hurt I had the option to push on or quit. When I experienced severe abdominal discomfort and diarrhea from my Crohn's attacks, I didn't have any option but to let the symptoms take their course. The lack of control was the most uncomfortable feeling of all.

It took a lot of work to train and raise money for the kids' camp but it seemed like a noble goal. This disease is something chronic that affects everyone differently, and I am no exception. I've certainly had my fair share of discomfort over the past 20 years, but only two serious attacks. As uncomfortable as things were for me at times, I felt pretty darn lucky I wasn't in and out of the hospital every other week, having surgery, or shooting steroids like some of the kids I've met.

For a while, I was deceived and thought I had the disease under control. Perhaps my healthy lifestyle and good living were the reason I wasn't affected for such a long time. But when I was hospitalized last year, feelings that seemed to be part of a different life started coming back to me. The worst part wasn't the pain, or the drugs, or the diarrhea, but the helplessness. I was stuck in a room and told I couldn't go anywhere and I couldn't do anything. I had to lie in bed all day surrounded by a sterile environment that reeked of illness and depression. That was the worst feeling for me, and perhaps the feeling that pushed me towards running.

When I ran fast my adrenaline flowed, the world rushed by, and the scenery changed. I felt my blood pumping through my veins and all of my senses became stimulated. My body was working too hard and too long to experience any of this so-called "irritable bowel disease" and I finally felt like I could take control of my pain.

For the first time since last year's attack, I felt freedom and I couldn't get enough of it. In fact, that's how ultra-running evolved for me in the first place: 5k's became 10k's, and 10k's became marathons, and marathons became 50 milers, and 50 milers became longer. The more time I spent on the trail, the more control I had, the more freedom I experienced. Like many other distance runners, as my strength grew I felt like I could go on forever.

When I first set out to run across Morocco, I had 10 years of competitive ultra-running under my belt. I had placed in the top 10 percent of numerous ultra-marathons and trained often. I enjoyed the camaraderie of the sport and the edge of competition. I befriended people like myself that had a passion for running and the outdoors. Even though their motives may not have been the same as my own, we connected. I felt that I had found my place in the world and could come close to competing on more of a professional level. I was physically and psychologically stronger than ever before. With the exception of the occasional bowel discomfort, which I rationalized everyone experienced, I was unstoppable and my Crohn's was twenty years behind me.

Maybe I had to suffer another serious attack so I could remember exactly who I was and what I was made of. And when it hit, it hit hard, and tore me down both physically and mentally. During my weekend in the hospital I lost almost fifteen pounds and rode a roller coaster of intense drugs ranging from anti-coagulants to morphine. Some of these I would continue to take during my very slow, long healing process over the next four months. Eventually, I would be put on a mild anti-inflammatory that would be prescribed for the rest of my life.

All of this made me remember, and it made me

wonder how kids or people with the same illness make it through their lives having to deal with this every few years or every few months. It made me question if I had been psychologically and physically strong enough to avoid hospitalization all of those years, or whether I was just lucky enough to dodge so many bullets for such a long time.

After leaving the hospital last year, I needed help. First and foremost, I had to help myself back to the athlete I once was because that was my identity and I felt naked without it. It took a long time. I relied on the love and support of family and friends to get me back on the trail. I slowly progressed over a few months, fell into my regular training routines, and started racing again. It was hard to justify my race times as I ran them so much faster in the past. I often wondered when I could stop rationalizing my performance with the phrase "I'm still recovering from my hospitalization." Eventually my performance improved, but only one race would put my mind to rest—the one that was taken away from me when I was hospitalized. By committing to the upcoming Marathon des Sables, I outlined a goal that would put me back into a positive state of health, both physically and mentally.

As I prepared for the race, it dawned on me that I had the opportunity to help others while helping myself. I decided to raise money for a camp that would allow kids to spend time with peers suffering from the same illness. Because of my last attack, I had been put in contact with many people who had the same chronic illness. It seemed everyone had his or her own story of success or failure with the disease. A camp would allow kids the opportunity to learn about themselves and their disease, instead of forcing them to struggle through their teen years as I had.

As a kid, I understood very little about my disease. All I knew was that I didn't feel well. As I grew older and made it through more doctors' visits with less probing, I distanced myself further from my disease. I built a wall of ignorance to protect myself from any memories of my childhood hospitalization. Eventually, the wall crashed down and, as a responsible adult, I had to face Crohn's. If this camp could keep one kid from building that wall, I felt it would be worth the whole race. As I raced across the sands of the Moroccan desert, these were the thoughts that drove me forward every step of the way.

In actuality, my time across the desert turned out to be one of the most testing weeks of my life. So testing, that at one point I thought long and hard about my last visit to the hospital and wondered how it could have been so much worse. I realized I might have underestimated the power of Mother Nature when comparing her to the discomfort of a hospital room. I wondered if I had indeed cursed myself.

The only thing that made this painful event simplistic in comparison to dealing with my Crohn's was that it was supposed to be a voluntary act of discomfort. After raising so many pledges for the kids' camp, one thing pushed me forward: I kept picturing myself not completing the event. There would be no swimming, no capture the flag, no games of checkers, no camp where children could connect with each other. I envisioned people backing out on their pledges and saying, "Yes Michael, I know we pledged 100 dollars, but you promised to complete this race in Morocco. Since you didn't stick to your end of the deal, I really don't think we should have to stick to ours."

In spite of the worst weather in over ten years, with sandstorms of epic proportions, I was able to push through my misery and "capture my own flag" to complete the event.

As I tell the story over and over to friends, relatives, and the many generous sponsors, it takes on more clarity for me. It's clear that this fund-raising event was a difficult endeavor that I chose to take on. Crohn's, on the other hand, is not something I've chosen, and it continues to challenge me. With both running and Crohn's, I get to choose how positively or negatively I face them.

Looking over at my tattered shoes I remember how they brought me so much pleasure. I also remember why I run: because in spite of some of "the toughest footraces" I've already won, I know there will always be tougher ones down the road. Running reminds me to enjoy life while I can, even when I have to lace up and run in the rain.

Step by Step

Karen Myers

There are 26 stairs leading up to my friend Marie's apartment, where I have been invited to dinner. Marie is the best cook I know. She makes chili and rhubarb pie and chocolate chip cookies. But she lives on the top floor of her building.

I open Marie's front gate, which is interlaced with the flowering white buds of a potato vine. I know that it is a potato vine only because I planted three of them in my front yard two years ago. One of them is dead, but the other two are thriving.

Eight steps across the gray cement entryway and I begin my ascent. The first time I visited Marie I thought I might have to drop the workshop she was hosting—there was too little parking and too many stairs. The sidewalk was slick with rain, and the climb to her front door felt like a trek up Mount Everest.

I start with my left foot, the stronger of my legs. My left calf is shapely and rounded, like a woman who has grown up climbing hills. My right calf has become withered and thin, blotches of sunken skin where muscle should be. My massage therapist says if I walk barefoot on the beach it will help build up those muscles. I hope he is right.

I purposefully pound my white canvas sneakers on top of each black-checkered stair, creating a thumping noise, as though I'm trying to squish a cockroach. I wear sneakers that are light because the weight of a heavy shoe feels like something more to carry, another burden for my muscles to absorb. My friend, Andrew, who also has muscular dystrophy, says that high-top sneakers help steady his walk. But the last time I saw him he was having trouble getting up the slope of a curb.

The slap of sole to cement makes me feel more grounded, more in touch with my lower limbs. Too often I float in my mind, far away from the prison of my body, far away from the tightness in my hip joints and the fatigue in my legs. Stomping my feet on the ground draws me down into my body and I feel strong and powerful and fierce.

I lift my thighs as high as they go, trying to bring them somewhere near my chest. I can barely lift them to my stomach. But still, I can lift them. I'm stronger than most of the people who attend my muscular dystrophy support groups. I remember the former firefighter who looked up at me from his wheelchair and said, "God, I wish I could move like you."

The mental game begins: I will not touch the iron handrail. This would be to give in—to the disease, to my weakness. Soon my body would forget what it has been able to do. I cannot let it forget. My shoulders sway to the left, then to the right with each step, my upper body compensating for the weakness of my pelvis and gluteus medius. Before Dr. Schmidt diagnosed me, when I was 13, I didn't know where the gluteus medius muscle was. He said muscular dystrophy is degenerative, that I should stay active but "don't overdo it." Every year I go to his office and he pushes against my arms and asks me to flex my ankles and walk on my toes. Then he marks numbers in my medical file and tells me to come back next year.

I will not grab the handrail. It's right there, to my left. It would be so easy to reach out and touch its cold green metal. I could pull myself up a bit and steady my gait. But I need to practice balance for those times at the movies when there isn't a handrail to support me—like when I went with my niece to one of those new stadium-style theaters.

I reach the platform between the second and third floors and rest at the doormat that says "Welcome." I try to keep the momentum going, but fatigue has settled in. My body slows down, as though I'm walking through a fog of thick humidity. I remember heavy summer days when the heat felt like a child clinging to my legs. That sensation assaults me now, even though the air is cool. My thighs fill with lead. My right foot lands on its outer rim. Did I used to walk more flat-footed? Is this the first sign that my ankles are becoming weaker?

Only one more flight, I tell myself. The corridor is dark and winds to the right. I can do this. One, two, three, four . . . I count in my head to distract myself from the effort of my body. I don't know when I started counting steps. Maybe four or five years ago when a stroll to the corner store became a series of calculated movements. One step in front of the other, heel, toe, heel, toe.

I reach Marie's apartment. It smells of chili and garlic bread. Marie bounces toward me and throws open her arms. I am short of breath when she hugs me hello. I smile and lean into her shoulder.

"Hey, look! No hands!" This is what I used to scream to my brother when I could still ride a bicycle. Today I climbed Marie's 26 stairs—and I didn't touch the hand-rail.

Contributors

Raymond J. Aguilera can often be found chasing his Jack Russell Terrier around the San Francisco Bay Area. When he's not at the dog park, he's busy as the managing editor of *Bent: A Journal of Cripgay Voices.* His writing and other nonsense can be found at RayAguilera.com.

Riua Akinshegun—visual artist, writer, and performance artist—follows the advice of her creative muse: "Don't worry about growing old, worry about staying new." She has performed her poetry and stories for the Armand Hammer Museum, the Mark Taper Forum's Other Voices, the Writers Guild of America, and the Maafa Conference in Brooklyn, New York, as well as on international stages of Mexico, Guyana, and Suriname. She has exhibited her art in Guyana, Mali, Nigeria, and the U.S., and she conducts workshops on art as a healing process. *The Most Mutinous Leapt Overboard,* her interactive installation on the Middle Passage (trans-Atlantic slave trade), became the inspiration for S. Pearl Sharp's documentary film, *The Healing Passage: Voices From the Water,* which premiered in June 2004. She has just completed *Market Bag,* a family story, and is currently working on her autobiography, *Home Grown.* Riua Akinshegun has been wheelchair-mobile since the 1970's, the result of a bullet that left her a paraplegic, incomplete (L2-L5).

Marguerite Bouvard is the author of four books of poetry and several nonfiction books, including *The Path Through Grief: A Compassionate Guide.* Her latest book is *Prayers for Comfort in Difficult Times* (Wind Publications, 2004). She has been a scholar at the Women's Studies Research Center at Brandeis University since illness caused her to quit her job as a professor. She has been battling interstitial cystitis and fibromyalgia for the past 15 years. During this time, she has published a number of books on human rights, including *Revolutionizing Motherhood: The Mothers of the Plaza de Mayo* and *Women Reshaping Human Rights: How Extraordinary Women Are Changing the World.*

Lawrence Bradby was born in Scotland in 1968 and took a degree in geology in Norwich, England. After working for several years as a researcher, he became ill with M.E. (myalgic encephalomyelitis, also called chronic fatigue syndrome). First the field trips to glaciers were cancelled, then the lab work, and finally he was bed-bound, too weak to hold up a book, with nothing but howling tinnitus and tropical headaches for company. During this period he began to write poetry. His poems have appeared in various magazines, including *The Rialto, The Reater, Reactions, Pretext, PN Review,* and *Iambosaurus.* He has published four booklets, all with Sideline Publications: *Breathe In Conk Out* (2001), *The Best Bloody Job in the World* (2002), *Bookmark Book* (2003), and *Sweep and Veer* (2005). In 2003 he completed his M.A. in Creative Writing at the University of East Anglia. Lawrence has an ongoing interest in alternative ways to put poetry into the public domain.

Rev. Hugh Burns, O.P., is a Catholic priest of the Dominican Order. A native of Boston, Fr. Burns now resides in Pleasantville, NY. Ordained in 1982, he has worked in Hispanic ministry in Washington and was Director of Formation for the Dominican Friars in Puerto Rico. Since 1989 he has been preaching and conducting seminars throughout the United States and the Caribbean. Fr. Burns is also a writer whose commentaries on religious issues are heard on National Public Radio's *Morning Edition.* His humorous essays are also broadcast in the New York area on public radio. His radio essay, "The Fruitcake," received an award from Public Radio News Directors Inc. (PRNDI). Other essays have been published in various Catholic periodicals. Fr. Burns has been living with alopecia universalis since 1986. It is an autoimmune disorder that kills the hair follicles–in his case all of them. The noted wig still lies in its unopened box.

Josh Danoff moved back to his hometown of Amherst, Massachusetts, after graduating from college and started a dry-stack stonemasonry company. He owned and operated it for five years before contracting Lyme disease. He has since been a featured writer on the companion DVD to Pat Schneider's *Writing Alone and with Others* and has lived in Melbourne, Australia, where he was a freelance writer for the venture capital magazine *Australia Anthill.* In addition to Australia, he has traveled extensively throughout Southeast Asia, New Zealand, Costa Rica, and Ireland. He lives in Amherst, where he is an elementary school special education teacher.

Pierre Delattre's career as an artist has run parallel with a career as a writer. He began as a graphic artist in 1971, doing the cover painting and 17 illustrations for his first novel, *Tales of a Dalai Lama,* and has done the jacket painting for two other books. He has worked as contributing editor and lead essayist on art for *THE,* Santa Fe's Monthly Magazine of the Arts. His books include *Walking on Air, Episodes,* and *Woman on the Cross.* For more information on his paintings and writings, visit his website at www.pierredelattre.com.

Varda Nowack Goldstein wrote "My Visualization" in 2001-2002 while battling advanced breast cancer. Subsequent to a mastectomy, Varda developed a brain tumor, which was removed in June 2003. This left Varda functioning at only about 25% of her usual self. After a couple of months, the doctors discovered that the breast cancer had metastasized into the spinal fluid. Varda wasn't in any pain and was well-loved and supported by her family and friends. At her request, her family and friends were partaking of Rosh Hashanah dinner when she took her last breath at the stroke of 7:00 p.m. on September 26, 2003, the eve of the Jewish New Year. Her devoted husband, Imron, remains her biggest fan.

Laban Carrick Hill was a 2004 National Book Award Finalist for his *Harlem Stomp! A Cultural History of the Harlem Renaissance,* which received more than 25 awards and honors. His young adult novel *Casa Azul* is a New York Public Library Book of the Teen Age 2006 selection. He has written more than twenty books for children, young adults, and adults.

Molly Ivins was a progressive political commentator, journalist, and author based in Austin, Texas. She was a syndicated columnist with nationwide distribution; her column appeared in over 300 newspapers across the United States. Her articles appeared in *Esquire, The Atlantic Monthly, The Nation, Harper's, The Progressive, The Progressive Populist,* and *Mother Jones.* She had been a commentator for NPR, *The News Hour with Jim Lehrer,* and *60 Minutes.* Her recent books include *Who Let the Dogs In?: Incredible Political Animals I Have Known* (Random House, 2004) and *Bushwhacked: Life in George W. Bush's America* with Lou Dubose (Random House, 2003). She died in 2007 after battling inflammatory breast cancer.

Maggie Jochild received the Loving Lesbians Poetry Award from the Astraea Lesbian Writer's Fund in both 2002 and 2005. She is a sixth-generation Texan, mother, grandmother, and godmother who earns her living as a medical transcriptionist. For four years she was a core writing and performing member of Actual Lives, a theater troupe for disabled artists, directed by Terry Galloway. For six years her work has been published in *Di-Verse-City Anthology,* the Austin International Poetry Festival anthology. Other recent publications include *Natural Bridge, Texas Poetry Calendar 2006, Voices of Racial Justice Anthology, Asphodel,* and *Rockhurst Review.* She has been a workshop programmer for *Finding Voice Productions,* coordinated by Sharon Bridgforth. Her disabilities include lifelong moderate-to-severe asthma, bilateral bony deformities of both tibia and feet, and polycystic ovary disease. She was raised poor white trash and came out as a lesbian at age nine in 1965, the same year she started writing poetry. She writes because, as Anne Lamott says, it will kill her if she does not.

Deborah Kent grew up in Little Falls, New Jersey, where she became the first totally blind student to attend the local public school. She received a B.A. in English from Oberlin College and a master's degree from Smith College School for Social Work. After working for four years at University Settlement House on New York's Lower East Side, she decided to pursue her lifelong interest in writing. The town of San Miguel de Allende, with its thriving community of expatriate writers and artists, became her home for the next five years. In San Miguel she completed her first young-adult novel, *Belonging*. While there, she also met her husband, children's author R. Conrad (Dick) Stein. For the past twenty years she has lived in Chicago, where she continues to write both fiction and nonfiction. She is also an active member of the National Federation of the Blind. Her daughter Janna, whose birth inspired the essay in this collection, has graduated from college and is currently working as a teacher's aide with teens with disabilities.

Jennifer Kern has worn several hats since she sustained a spinal cord injury in 1985. Professionally, she has worked as a teacher, attorney, disability advocate, wheelchair builder, fundraiser, and public speaker, and has led projects in five developing countries. She currently studies East-West psychology in San Francisco and hopes to integrate the various hats some day. She lives in Berkeley, California, with her son Jasper, who at nineteen months loves to say "apple," and her beloved cat Strix.

Donna Kichner holds an M.S. in Secondary Education English from Bloomsburg University in Pennsylvania. Starting in 1969, she taught in public schools and remained in the teaching profession until her retirement in 2001. Donna suffered a life-threatening stroke at the age of twenty-five resulting from a strep infection that was not completely cleared up. She recovered quite handily from this first stroke to lead a full life as a wife, mother, teacher, and youth worker. Then, in 1997, she suffered a second more debilitating stroke and, in 1998, fractured her left (stronger) ankle. Besides accomplishing her daily living skills, she is presently trying to fill her days with rewarding activities such as counted cross stitching, volunteer GED tutoring, and literacy tutoring.

Barbara Lehmann became an actress at the University of California, Berkeley, after being treated successfully for Hodgkin's disease in 1968 at the age of thirteen. Because her beautiful performances were so moving, she was cast in lead roles at the Shakespeare Festival in Boulder, Colorado, and in modern plays at the Berkeley Repertory Theater. In the late 1980s, she moved to New York to try her luck at a career in acting. Living in the East Village, she turned to performance art, worked at the Franklin Furnace, and took her performances to Europe. During this time, she also wrote fashion articles for *The Village Voice*. After staging the trauma of her adolescent illness, she began to write about her year of treatment at Stanford Hospital in 1968. Before she was able to finish her fact-based novel, *Glowing in the Dark,* she died suddenly in 1993 at the age of 37.

Erin Lewy is a writer, editor, teacher, and activist who believes strongly in the power of words, spoken and written, to create social and personal change. The story included in this anthology began with an image of the characters, who insisted they would settle for no less than a novel. She is currently working on the first of what she hopes will become a series of young-adult titles confronting issues of disability, autonomy, identity, and sexuality. A later version of this story appeared in *Breath and Shadow: A Journal of Disability Culture and Literature* (June 2004), at www. abilitymaine.org/breath.

Dustin Michael suffers from severe allergy- and exercise-induced asthma, a condition made more dangerous by his absentmindedness and his enjoyment of physical activity. He is a writer for the news bureau of Southeast Missouri State University and has been published in *Journey Literary Magazine* and *Rain Taxi.*

N.M. Moro resides outside of Ithaca, New York with her partner and two cat-kids. She holds a B.A. in English from Wells College, and an M.A. in Creative Writing from Binghamton University. Her work has been published in several literary anthologies, including *The Healing Muse,* edited by the late Bonnie St. Andrews; *I'm Home* (2005), edited by Ann Wells; and the Lambda-nominated anthology *Hot and Bothered 4: Short Fiction on Lesbian Desire (2003),* edited by Karen Tulchinsky. She is currently writing a memoir.

Madeleine Parish writes about spiritual growth and moral dilemmas in both fiction and non-fiction. Her novel *The Geography Lesson* was recognized in the 2004 PEN Women of San Francisco competition. *A Pilgrim's Way* is her collection of meditations for people recovering from chronic illness. Her short fiction and essays appear in periodicals (including *The Phoenix* and *Christianity and the Arts*) and anthologies. A graduate of Cornell University, she was an award-winning corporate communications executive before being diagnosed with CFIDS in 1995. She lives and writes in Fairfield County, CT, where she helps plan the annual Festival of Words.

Clint Pearson, M.D. is a practicing family physician, a former rock climber, and a former long-distance runner who battles multiple sclerosis on a daily basis. Fortunately, he has help from Ursula, his lovely wife of twenty years, and the two have been blessed with twins, Denali and Jasmine, now four years old. Today they all reside amidst the beautiful Redwoods outside of Crescent City, California. Drawing upon his experience as a physician and as a multiple sclerosis patient, Clint has spent over ten years writing *Falling* and is hoping to publish the work soon.

Michael Raymond, Ph.D. is a professor of English at Stetson University. Diagnosed with Type I diabetes in 1955, he is the author of *The Human Side of Diabetes* (1992), *A Guidebook for Diabetes Self-Care* (1993), *The Language Arts/Computer Book* (1984), and *MEW: More Effective Writing* (1980), as well as articles, stories, and essays on a wide range of topics. Married for 38 years with two grown sons, Mike has been a double amputee living in a wheelchair since 2001.

Glenn "Omodiende" Reitz is currently finishing a Ph.D. in African American Studies at Temple University, after medically retiring from a career in the United States Navy. His poetic and visual works on race, sexuality, and AIDS have been published in Temple's graduate series, *Schuylkill.* As a guest lecturer he discusses "Living with Dying"—having been living with AIDS for more than 17 years. His symptoms include wasting, constant pain, fatigue, and indirect problems including brain lesions and retina damage, in addition to bouts of shingles and PCP pneumonia. To view his poems and artwork, visit his website at http://astro.temple.edu/~greitz.

Rachel Naomi Remen, M.D. is Clinical Professor of Family and Community Medicine at UCSF School of Medicine and the Founder and Director of the Institute for the Study of Health and Illness at Commonweal. She is one of the pioneers of Holistic and Integrative Medicine and the Founder and Director of the Healer's Art curriculum for medical students, which is now being taught in more than one third of medical schools nationwide. She is co-founder and medical director of the Commonweal Cancer Help Program, one of the first support groups for cancer patients in America, featured in the groundbreaking 1993 Bill Moyer's PBS series *Healing and the Mind.* Dr. Remen's bestselling books *Kitchen Table Wisdom: Stories that Heal* and *My Grandfather's Blessings: Stories of Strength, Refuge and Belonging* (Riverhead Press) have been published in 18 languages.

Marcy Sheiner is the author of *Perfectly Normal: A Mother's Memoir,* available at www.iUniverse.com

or via her website: www.marcysheiner.tripod.com. Her fiction and essays have been published in numerous anthologies, most recently *The Essential Hip Mama: Writing from the Cutting Edge of Parenting,* edited by Ariel Gore. Her stories have also appeared on the websites *Pulse* and *Slow Trains,* and she has edited a dozen anthologies of women's erotic fiction. In 2002 she was diagnosed with COPD (Chronic Obstructionary Pulmonary Disease) and was hospitalized seven times until she was stabilized.

Floyd Skloot's memoir of living with viral-caused brain damage, *In the Shadow of Memory* (Nebraska, 2003), won the PEN Center USA Literary Award in Creative Nonfiction, the Independent Publishers Book Award in Creative Nonfiction, and was a finalist for both the PEN Award for the Art of the Essay and the Barnes & Noble Discover Award. The sequel, *A World of Light* (Nebraska, 2005), was a *New York Times Book Review* Editors' Choice selection. His fourth collection of poems, *Approximately Paradise* (Tupelo Press, 2005), won a Pacific Northwest Booksellers Book Award, and his fifth collection, *The End of Dreams* (LSU Press, 2006), has just been published. His work has been included in *The Best American Essays, The Best American Science Writing, The Art of the Essay, The Best Spiritual Writing,* and *The Pushcart Prize Anthology.*

Merry Speece has published two chapbooks of poetry and has been a recipient of a state arts commission fellowship in prose. Her *Sisters Grimke Book of Days* was published in 2003 by Oasis Books (England). Work of hers is included in the anthologies *Nixon Under the Bodhi Tree and Other Works of Buddhist Fiction* and *I Have* *a Song for It: Modern Poems of Ohio.* She has spent most of her life in rural Ohio. For more than twenty-five years she has been ill with what was finally diagnosed in 1990 as chronic fatigue immune dysfunction syndrome.

Ryan G. Van Cleave's most recent books include a poetry collection, *The Magical Breasts of Britney Spears* (Red Hen Press, 2006), and a creative writing textbook, *Contemporary American Poetry: Behind the Scenes* (Allyn & Bacon/Longman, 2003). He lives in upstate South Carolina. He inherited his susceptibility to migraines from his mother.

Sharon Wachsler likes to mix and match her media and genres: her essays and cartoons have been published in the U.S. and abroad (including translation into German); her fiction is in over a dozen books; her articles appear in numerous magazines, papers, and journals. Notable achievements include a Pushcart nomination and Peregrine Prize for poetry, consecutive years of publication in the *Best American Erotica* series, and founding and editing *Breath & Shadow* (www.abilitymaine.org/breath), the only literary journal written exclusively by people with disabilities. Sharon is best known for her Sick Humor cartoons and essays about life with disability, which she is compiling into a book, *Sick Humor: Full Frontal Disability.* To check out her cartoon postcards visit www. sickhumorpostcards.com. To learn about her writing classes, go to www.sharonwachsler.com.

Caitlin M. Warde is a writer who will be pursuing her M.F.A. in fiction at the University of North Carolina at Wilmington this fall. She has been disabled since 1999 with Crohn's disease. Despite extreme fatigue and severe daily pain, she writes at least one page a day. She is supported by her wonderful partner, Eileen, and her schnoodle, Maggie.

Patricia Wellingham-Jones, Ph.D., RN, is a former psychology researcher/writer/editor/lecturer who has turned to writing short stories and poetry. Her work has been published in numerous anthologies, journals, and Internet magazines, including *Mšbius, Midwest Poetry Review, Liberty Hill Poetry Review, Red River Review, Edgz,* and *Niederngasse.* She won the Reuben Rose International Poetry Prize (Israel) in 2003. Two spinal surgeries, neck and lumbar, left her with dysfunction and chronic pain. She is also a 5-year survivor of breast cancer, yet seldom writes about these issues, preferring to capture life in all its madness as it happens around her. However, one of her ten poetry chapbooks is *Don't Turn Away: Poems About Breast Cancer,* in its third printing and given out by Reach To Recovery volunteers. Her website is www.wellingham-jones.com.

Michael Wille was diagnosed with Crohn's disease at the age of 13. Michael holds an A.O.S. from the Culinary Institute of America and a B.A. in Journalism from San Francisco State University. He is a chef-instructor at the Professional Culinary Institute and has just written his first cookbook, *Discovering Authentic Mexican Cooking,* featuring the recipes of Berkeley's famed Dona Tomas

Restaurant. Michael lives an active life in the hills of Los Gatos, CA, hiking and running with his wife and son. He is an active member of the Crohn's and Colitis Foundation of America, striving to prove to other children—as well as himself—that Crohn's disease should not affect the richness of life, but only enhance its complexities.

Adan Williams is an educator, world traveler, non-denominational minister, and artist. He graduated from UCLA's writing program in 1983. While at UCLA, he published articles, poetry, illustrations, and short stories in campus reviews and papers. He currently resides in Southern California.

About the Editors

Felicia Ferlin lives with thoracic outlet syndrome from a repetitive strain injury (RSI). She holds a M.A. in Professional Writing from Carnegie Mellon University in her hometown of Pittsburgh, Pennsylvania. Prior to her computer-use injury, she produced and contributed to numerous on-line and hard-copy manuals, articles, and technical documents for organizations such as IBM, Carnegie Mellon University, and the National Science Foundation Network. She currently works part-time as a therapeutic swim coach helping other RSI patients learn how to rehabilitate themselves through aerobic conditioning.

Karen Myers is a freelance writer who lives in San Francisco, California. Her work has been published in numerous newspapers, magazines, and anthologies, including *The Plain Dealer Sunday Magazine, Magical Blend, The Philadelphia Inquirer,* and *2Do Before I Die.* She is a member of the board of the Self-Healing Research Foundation, which oversees The School for Self-Healing. At the age of 13, she was diagnosed with facioscapulohumeral (FSH) dystrophy, the third most common form of muscular dystrophy.

Acknowledgements

"The Café Lady" by Raymond J. Aguilera originally appeared in *BENT: A Journal of Cripgay Voices*, which can be found at www.bentvoices.org.

"The Joy of Polio," copyright 1993, by Pierre Delattre is reprinted from *Episodes* with the permission of Graywolf Press, Saint Paul, Minnesota.

"My Visualization" by Varda Nowack Goldstein is printed by permission of her estate.

"A Grateful Cancer Survivor" by Molly Ivins is reproduced with permission of the *Star-Telegram*. Copyright © 2000 *Star-Telegram*. All rights reserved. Any unauthorized reproduction of this article is strictly prohibited. For reprint information contact the *Star-Telegram* at 817-390-7573.

"Somewhere a Mockingbird" by Deborah Kent originally appeared in the anthology *Bigger than the Sky: Disabled Women on Parenting*, edited by Michele Wates and Rowen Jade and published by The Women's Press, London, in 1999.

Barbara Lehmann's excerpt from *Glowing in the Dark* is reprinted by permission of her estate.

"Crohn's Disease" by Rachel Naomi Remen, M.D. is reprinted by permission of the author from *Wounded Healers: A Book of Poems by People Who Have Had Cancer and Those Who Love Them*, which is edited by Rachel Naomi Remen, M.D. (Wounded Healer Press, 1994).

The excerpt from *Perfectly Normal: A Mother's Memoir* by Marcy Sheiner (People With Disability Press, 2002) is reprinted by permission of the author.

The work "Sick" by Merry Speece was first published in *Quarter After Eight: A Journal of Prose and Commentary,* Volume 10, 2004.

"Pap Goes the Wheezer" by Sharon Wachsler first appeared in *Sojourner,* March 2001.

www.ingramcontent.com/pod-product-compliance
Lightning Source LLC
LaVergne TN
LVHW091048080826
845145LV00002B/671